MAYO CLINIC

ESSENTIAL GUIDE TO

PROSTATE HEALTH

Lance A. Mynderse, M.D.

Medical Editor-in-Chief

Mayo Clinic
Rochester, Minnesota

Published by Mayo Clinic Health Solutions

For bulk sales to employers, member groups and health-related companies, contact Mayo Clinic Health Solutions, 200 First St. SW, Rochester, MN, 55905, or send an e-mail to *SpecialSalesMayoBooks@Mayo.edu.*

Address inquiries to Mayo Clinic Health Solutions, Permissions Department, 200 First St., SW, Fifth floor Centerplace Building, Rochester, MN, 55905.

Stock photography from Artville, BananaStock, Brand X Pictures, Comstock, Corbis, Creatas, Digital Stock, Digital Vision, EyeWire, Food Shapes, Image Ideas, © Isabelle Rozenbaum/PhotoAlto, Photodisc, Rubberball and Stockbyte. The individuals pictured are models, and the photos are used for illustrative purposes only. There's no correlation between the individuals portrayed and the conditions or subjects being discussed. The photos on page 133 are courtesy of Intuitive Surgical Inc.

Library of Congress Control Number: 2008934187

Printed in Canada

First Edition

1 2 3 4 5 6 7 8 9 10

About Mayo Clinic

Mayo Clinic evolved from the frontier practice of Dr. William Worrall Mayo and the partnership of his two sons, Drs. William J. and Charles H. Mayo, in the early 1900s. Pressed by the demands of their busy practice in Rochester, Minn., the Mayo brothers invited other physicians to join them, pioneering the private group practice of medicine. Today, with more than 2,000 physicians and research scientists at major locations in Rochester, Minn., Jacksonville, Fla., and Phoenix and Scottsdale, Ariz., Mayo Clinic is dedicated to providing comprehensive diagnoses, accurate answers, and effective treatments.

With this depth of medical knowledge, experience and expertise, Mayo Clinic occupies an unparalleled position as a health information resource. Since 1983, Mayo Clinic has published reliable health information for millions of consumers through a variety of award-winning newsletters, books and online services. Revenue from these publishing activities supports Mayo Clinic programs, including medical education and medical research.

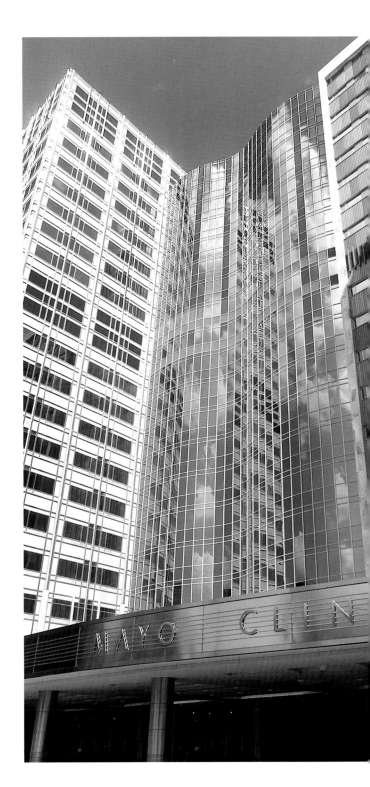

Editorial staff

Preface

For many adult males, the health concerns associated with prostate disease may be their first contact ever with a physician or, for that matter, with medical care. About 35 percent of men over age 50 will experience an inflammatory condition of the prostate known as prostatitis. Over 50 percent of men over age 60 will feel the discomfort of an enlarged prostate, or benign prostatic hyperplasia (BPH). Finally, prostate cancer is the most frequently diagnosed cancer — and the leading cause of cancer death — in American men.

Despite these sobering facts, prostate cancer, as well as other forms of prostate disease, is often easily treated, and the outlook for management, cure and survival is excellent. Advances in research, more sophisticated imaging technology and new medical procedures have enabled a much earlier diagnosis of prostate disease and more personalized treatment, reducing recovery time and avoiding many troublesome side effects.

This book will guide you, along with your spouse or significant other, through the decision process you may face as you work with your doctor to treat, manage and possibly cure prostate disease. The key to a good outcome is to educate yourself and to be involved with your doctor at an early stage to address your health concerns.

The more you know about prostate disease, the greater are your chances of identifying problems, making good decisions about treatment options and maintaining a high quality of life. Urologists, as key advocates for men's health, are in a position to educate, guide and assist all men with an individual-centered approach to the management of their health needs.

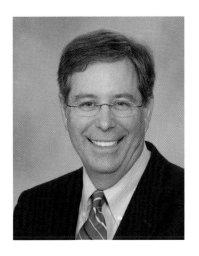

Lance A. Mynderse, M.D.
Medical Editor-in-Chief

Table of contents

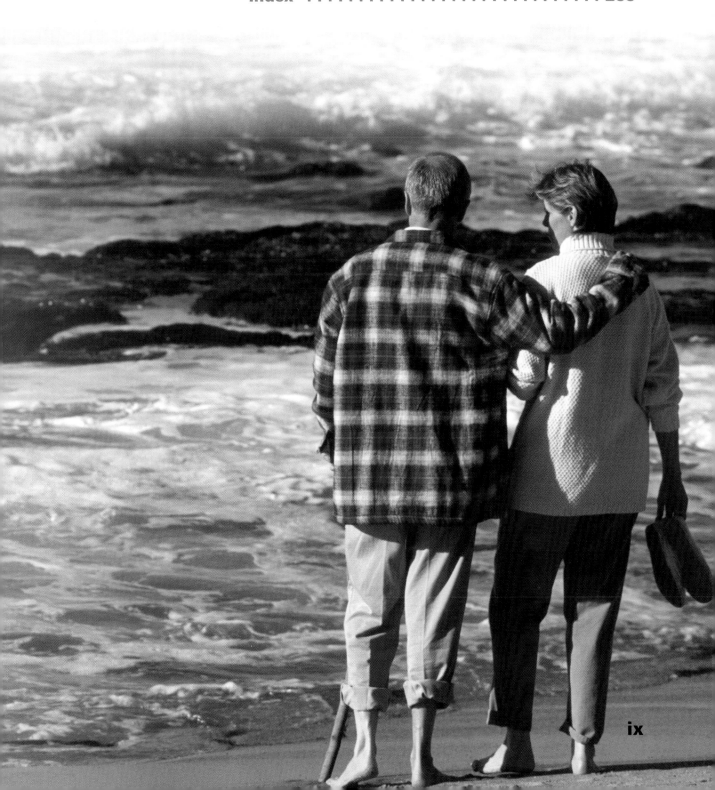

ix

Part 1

Prostate basics

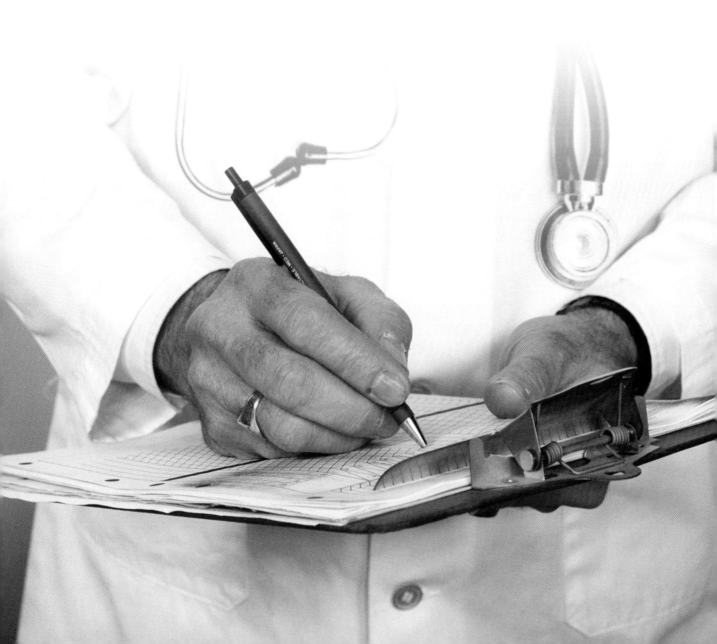

Chapter 1

About the prostate

The prostate gland can cause some of the most common health problems that men face, and cancer of the prostate is among the most feared. That's because prostate cancer, like breast cancer for women, often strikes at the core of human sexuality.

Beyond fear of cancer itself are the possible consequences of treatment — issues with bladder control (incontinence) and the inability to have an erection (erectile dysfunction). These problems can be as difficult to deal with as the cancer, eroding self-confidence and evoking feelings of lost masculinity.

But there's reason for optimism. If caught early, prostate cancer often can be successfully treated and cured.

Improved medical practice is reducing the risks of incontinence and erectile dysfunction. When these complications occur, treatment may limit their effects.

It's also important to understand that cancer isn't the only prostate problem. Inflammation and benign enlargement of the prostate are other common developments. Unlike cancer, these problems generally aren't life-threatening, but without treatment, they can become debilitating and painful.

Prostate problems are a fact of life for many men as they get older. However, with regular checkups, you can reduce your risk of serious disease and keep the condition from seriously disrupting your quality of life.

This book can help you better understand why prostate problems occur, identify symptoms early, and allow you to make informed decisions with your doctor regarding treatment.

Healthy prostate

Found only in men, the prostate gland lies at the base of the bladder, surrounding the urethra, the canal that provides an outlet for urine to exit from the bladder. Most of the prostate's outer surface is covered by a thin membrane called the capsule.

When you're born, the prostate is about the size of a pea. It continues to grow until you're about age 20, when it's roughly the size and shape of a walnut. The prostate gland remains this size until you're in your 40s, when it often starts to grow again. As you will learn, this second growth spurt is associated with prostate problems.

Treating the prostate can be difficult because the gland is bundled among many delicate organs, muscles, nerves and blood vessels. This is a reason why side effects such as bleeding, incontinence and erectile dysfunction are always a concern — for example, prostate surgery may affect the nerves leading to the penis, causing impotence.

The prostate gland plays a key role in the function of your reproductive system and — due to its location and to physical changes that may occur as you age — of your urinary system.

Reproductive system

The tiny glands in the peripheral and central zones of the prostate manufacture most of the fluid in semen. Tiny ducts carry this fluid to the urethra — the same channel that connects the bladder to your penis.

During orgasm, prostate fluid mixes with fluid from the seminal vesicles, located on each side of the prostate, and with sperm to form semen. Sperm travel up from your testicles through long tubes called the vasa deferentia (VA-suh def-uh-REN-shee-uh). Muscle contractions cause ejaculation, during which semen is propelled through the urethra and out of the penis.

To make sure semen doesn't move in the wrong direction and back up into the bladder, a ring of muscle at the neck of the bladder (internal sphincter)

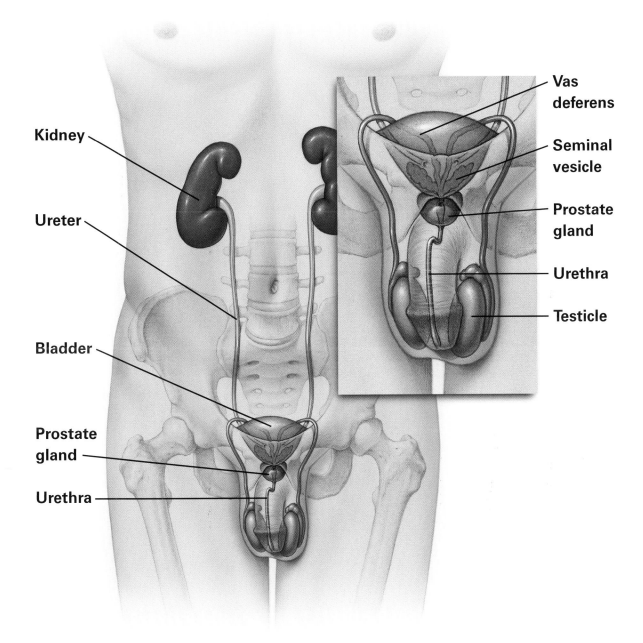

Kidney

Ureter

Bladder

Prostate
gland

Urethra

Vas
deferens

Seminal
vesicle

Prostate
gland

Urethra

Testicle

A central location

The prostate gland is tucked deep within the pelvic cavity, just below the bladder. Because of its location among so many organs, nerves, muscles and blood vessels, the prostate affects the health of both your reproductive system and urinary system.

A primer on basic prostate structure

The prostate gland consists of smooth muscle and spongy tissue containing thousands of tiny glands and ducts. Two major types of cells make up the organ. Epithelial cells are found in the glands. They secrete fluids that the body uses to produce semen — the fluid that transports and nourishes sperm. Stromal cells include connective tissue and smooth muscle that supports the epithelial cells.

The prostate produces an enzyme known as prostate-specific antigen (PSA). This enzyme is vital in the reproductive process because it helps break down semen once it has been delivered to a woman's vagina, allowing sperm to be freely mobile.

Three sections, or zones, of the prostate are separated by distinct structures and functions. The peripheral and central zones contain most of the prostate's glands, where semen fluid is produced. If prostate cancer develops, it's often in the peripheral zone and then spreads outward. The transitional zone, which surrounds the urethra in the center of the organ, is the part of your prostate that enlarges during the later growth stage that takes place in your 40s — exerting an inward pressure that can cause benign prostatic hyperplasia (BPH).

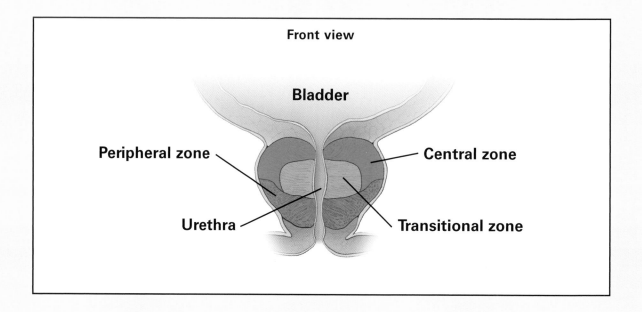

Front view

Bladder

Peripheral zone

Central zone

Urethra

Transitional zone

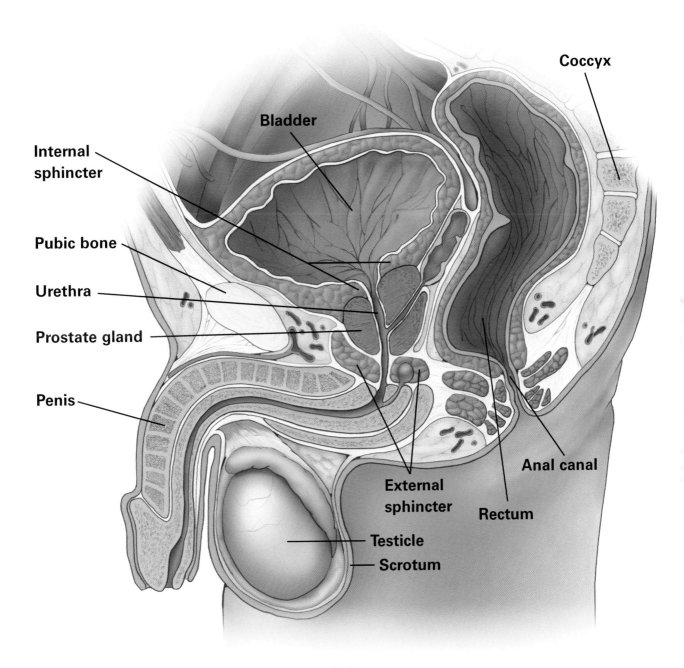

Coccyx

Bladder

Internal sphincter

Pubic bone

Urethra

Prostate gland

Penis

Anal canal

External sphincter

Rectum

Testicle

Scrotum

Cross-sectional view of the pelvic organs

The prostate gland surrounds the upper portion of the urethra, a narrow canal that provides a passage for urine leaving the bladder and for semen used for reproduction.

tightens during ejaculation, closing the urethra. The sphincter also keeps urine from discharging with the semen.

Urinary system

Although the prostate gland isn't a primary component of the urinary system, it's important to urinary health.

Your urinary system begins with your kidneys, which cleanse body fluids and produce urine. Urine travels from your kidneys to your bladder through long muscular tubes called ureters (u-REE-turs). Your bladder stores the urine until you urinate. During urination, the bladder muscle contracts and urine exits through the urethra to the penis.

Your prostate gland surrounds the top portion of the urethra, just below the bladder. Think of your prostate as a small apple with its core missing. The urethra runs through the missing core.

When your prostate is normal sized and healthy, this doesn't pose problems. But disease can develop in the prostate, causing tissue in this gland to swell or grow. This squeezes the urethra, making the channel narrow and affecting your ability to urinate.

When things go wrong

You aren't destined to develop prostate disease. Some men go through life without any prostate problems. Many, however, aren't so lucky. By the time they've become older adults, they experience some type of prostate problem. The symptoms may range from minor and mildly annoying to serious and painful.

Three different conditions commonly affect the prostate gland. Often, but not always, they can occur at different periods in a man's life.

Inflammation

Inflammation is the natural response of your body to infection or injury. Signs and symptoms often include redness, swelling and pain. Your prostate gland can swell and become tender at any age. Many times, a bacterial infection is the source of the inflammation. Other times, the cause of swelling and pain is unknown. Called prostatitis (pros-tuh-TIE-tis), prostate inflammation is the most common prostate problem among men under age 50.

Enlargement

Around age 45, tissue in your prostate gland often begins to grow again. This noncancerous growth is called benign prostatic hyperplasia (pros-TAT-ik hi-pur-PLA-zhuh), or BPH. It typically occurs in the transitional zone — the central portion of the gland.

The growth moves inward, causing prostate tissue to squeeze against the urethra and produce urinary problems. It's the most common prostate problem for men age 50 and older.

Cancer

According to the American Cancer Society, prostate cancer is the leading cause of cancer in American males. It most often occurs in men after age 50. The cancer results from abnormal and uncontrolled growth of tissue cells. Unlike BPH, cancer tumors generally develop in the outer part of the prostate, particularly in the peripheral zone.

Depending on the type of cancer, these tumors may grow very slowly or at a more rapid pace. Growth is generally outward, easily penetrating the thin membrane that encloses the prostate and spreading to surrounding tissue.

Estimated Male Cancer Cases United States, 2008

Total cases: 745,180
The urological cancers are highlighted.

Prostate	25%
Lung & bronchus	15%
Colon & rectum	10%
Urinary bladder	7%
Non-Hodgkin lymphoma	5%
Melanoma of skin	5%
Kidney & renal pelvis	4%
Oral cavity	3%
Leukemia	3%
Pancreas	3%
All other sites	20%

Source: American Cancer Society, 2008

Warning signs

Irritation or pain will often alert you to prostate problems. This is especially true of prostate inflammation or enlargement. Cancer typically provides less warning at an early stage.

The following signs and symptoms are often associated with prostate diseases. However, they aren't limited to the prostate. Other conditions, such as a urinary infections, can produce similar signs and symptoms:

- Urinating more frequently
- Excessive urination during the night (nocturia)
- Difficulty starting to urinate
- Decreased force in urine stream
- Interrupted flow of urine
- Dribbling after finishing urination
- Feeling as if your bladder isn't empty, even after urination
- Urgent need to urinate
- Blood in your urine (hematuria)
- Pain or burning sensation while urinating (dysuria)
- Painful ejaculation
- Tenderness or pain in the pelvis
- Persistent back or hip pain
- Pain or swelling in the testicles

Unfortunately, prostate cancer produces few, if any, symptoms in its early stages. It's not until later, when the disease is more difficult to treat, that symptoms such as urination difficulties or back pain may develop. That's why it's important to have regular prostate checkups to identify the disease early.

Are you at risk?

There's no simple formula that predicts who will encounter prostate problems. However, various factors — some of which you can control, others you can't — can affect your odds.

Uncontrollable factors

The most common risk factors for prostate disease may be the ones you can't control:

Age. As you get older, your risk of BPH and prostate cancer increases. It's estimated that more than half the men in the United States between the ages of 60 and 70 and as many as 90 percent between the ages of 70 and 90 exhibit signs and symptoms of BPH. Indeed, it may be that all men will have BPH if they live long enough.

The risk of prostate cancer also increases as men get older. More than 70 percent of men diagnosed with prostate cancer are age 65 or older.

Race and ethnicity. For reasons that aren't understood, black men are more likely to have prostate cancer than are men of any other group. They're also more likely to have prostate cancer at a younger age, and to develop an aggressive form of the disease.

Asian-American men, on the other hand, have the lowest rate of prostate cancer. The rate for Hispanic and American Indian men is lower than in whites. Black men have prostate cancer mortality rates about twice as high as white and Hispanic men, three times as high as Asian-Americans and five times as high as American Indian men.

Family history. Studies indicate that if your father or brother has prostate cancer, your risk of the disease is at least twice as great as that of the average American male. Depending on the number of relatives in your family with prostate cancer and the age at which they had it, your risk could be even higher. In families with a history of prostate cancer, the cancer generally occurs at a younger age.

Although age is the primary risk factor for BPH, family history also may play a role. Among men who have BPH in their 40s or early 50s, many carry an inherited gene that predisposes them to the disease. Just because you may carry the gene doesn't mean that the disease is inevitable — it simply increases your risk.

Bone mass. How much bone mass you have also may influence your risk of prostate cancer. Researchers at the Boston University School of Medicine found that in a group of about 1,000 men followed for about 30 years, those with the highest bone mass were more likely to develop prostate cancer than were men with the lowest amount of bone mass. The scientists concluded that bone mass may be one way to predict the likelihood of developing prostate cancer. The reasons behind the association weren't clear.

Controllable factors

The risk of prostate cancer varies among different populations. Because these differences don't appear to be genetic, researchers suspect that environment and lifestyle factors may play a role in your risk of prostate disease. However, at the moment, there are more questions about what these factors might be than about how you adapt or control them.

Sexual activity. Men with a history of sexually transmitted diseases (STDs) may be at higher risk of prostate cancer. In a review of 36 different studies that evaluated a possible link between STDs and prostate cancer, researchers found that men with a history of any STD were between 1.4 and 2.3 times as likely to develop prostate cancer as were men without such histories.

The number of sex partners that a man has had during his lifetime also may increase his risk of prostate cancer. One study concluded that men having two or more female partners during their teens, 20s, 40s and between the ages of 50 and 64 increased their risk of cancer.

The researchers also found that men who had 30 or more sexual partners in their lifetime had an increased risk of developing the more aggressive form of prostate cancer.

Environment. Researchers are studying whether exposure to certain substances at your job may play a role in increasing your risk. Higher death rates from prostate cancer can be found in certain blue-collar workers, such as farmers, mechanics, welders and industrial employees, than can be found in men in other occupations.

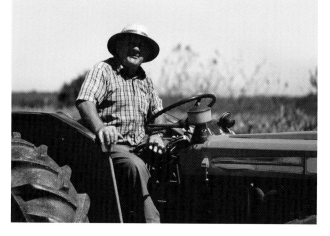

A Mayo Clinic study of more than 1,000 Iowa farmers found that those age 70 and older were about twice as likely to have prostate cancer as were nonfarmers of the same age. The study suggested that this increase may be due to occupational exposure — the identify of which was unclear — and not to dietary or lifestyle factors.

Diet. There's some evidence that a diet high in fat — particularly in saturated fat such as butter, lard and bacon fat — may increase your risk of prostate cancer. Researchers evaluated the diets of more than 50,000 health professionals over four years. They found that the men with high-fat diets were nearly twice as likely to have prostate cancer as were men who ate less fat.

The increased risk may be because fat increases production of the male sex hormone testosterone, which in turn speeds up the development of prostate cancer cells. If this theory proves correct, you may be able to reduce your risk of prostate cancer, or slow its development, simply by limiting the fat in your diet.

Several studies suggest that diets high in total calories may increase the risk of prostate cancer. A recent study has suggested that increased consumption of calcium and dairy products also raises your risk of prostate cancer.

On a more positive note, there's evidence that suggests chemicals found in soy products and certain vegetables and fruits may help lower your risk. See Chapter 11 for dietary steps that might protect you from prostate disease or delay its development.

Tobacco. Cigarette smoking may increase the risk of prostate cancer in younger men. In one study, researchers found that among men younger than 55 who'd had their prostate glands removed because of cancer, the current smokers were three times as likely as were the nonsmokers to have an advanced form of the disease.

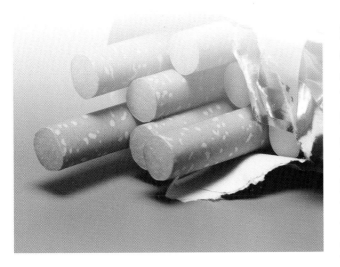

The researchers also found that the longer the men had smoked before being diagnosed, the more likely they were to have higher risk prostate cancer. Higher risk disease was defined as cancer that had spread beyond the prostate gland.

Supplemental hormones. Large doses of the nutritional supplement dehydroepiandrosterone (DHEA) may aggravate prostate enlargement or promote the development of prostate cancer. DHEA is a hormone that occurs naturally in your body. It's thought to be a precursor hormone — a chemical that's easily converted into other hormones, such as testosterone and estrogen. It's been shown that DHEA levels in your body increase sharply at puberty, peak during adulthood and then decrease gradually as you age.

DHEA supplements have been promoted to slow aging, burn fat, build muscle and strengthen the immune system. They're also touted as a treatment for illnesses such as Alzheimer's disease and Parkinson's disease. Research so far hasn't proved that the supplements provide these benefits. And in light of the relationship between DHEA and testosterone, long-term effects of supplement use requires further study.

Answers to your questions

Is it possible to be born with an abnormal prostate gland?

Yes. You can have a congenital abnormality in your prostate. Because of the prostate's location, men with congenital prostate abnormalities sometimes also have kidney abnormalities — affecting the function of both the urinary and reproductive systems. These conditions aren't common, however, and can easily be checked through X-ray or ultrasound images of the prostate gland and the kidneys.

I once had a sexually transmitted disease. Does this increase my risk of having prostate problems?

Possibly, yes. Some sexually transmitted diseases, such as gonorrhea and chlamydia, may cause inflammation in your urethra, the tube that carries urine out of your bladder. This inflammation can sometimes produce scar tissue that narrows or blocks the urethra, increasing your risk of infection of the lower urinary tract or infection in your prostate gland (prostatitis).

Is it true that a vasectomy can increase my risk of prostate cancer?

No. A few studies raised speculation that having a vasectomy may increase the risk of prostate cancer. However, researchers with the National Institutes of Health have reviewed data on vasectomies and concluded that the sterilization procedure doesn't increase a man's risk of getting prostate cancer.

Researchers believe that the questions raised in the studies can be explained by the fact that most vasectomies are done by urologists, and that men who have a good relationship with a urologist are more likely to get regular prostate checkups. Therefore, their cancer is detected earlier than that of men who don't get regular prostate examinations.

Chapter 2

Getting a prostate checkup

You are your own best protection against prostate disease. If you can help identify a prostate condition in its early stages, you have a better chance of successful treatment. How do you do that? By being aware of the signs and symptoms and scheduling regular checkups with your doctor.

There's no set schedule for prostate checkups. Every man has a different makeup and medical history. But if you're in your 40s or younger, an annual exam generally isn't necessary, unless you have a family history of prostate disease or you're experiencing prostate-related symptoms.

Age, however, is a major risk factor for prostate disease, and the older you are, the greater the likelihood of having problems with your prostate. Once you reach your 50s, you should consider scheduling an annual prostate examination with your doctor. And you should continue to have regular checkups throughout your lifetime.

What's involved in a typical exam varies, depending on your age, general health, medical history and lab test results from the previous checkup. Several tests may be performed, which are not conclusive by themselves but work well in combination.

Basic tests

Many doctors will include a prostate checkup as part of your regular physical examination. In addition to standard procedures and tests such as checking your blood pressure and listening to your heart and lungs, some or all of the following may be performed:

- Digital rectal examination
- Urinalysis
- Prostate-specific antigen test
- Ultrasound

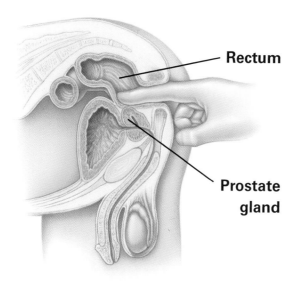

Rectum

Prostate gland

Digital rectal examination

During a digital rectal examination, your doctor inserts a gloved, lubricated finger into your rectum and feels the back wall of the prostate gland for enlargement, tenderness, lumps or hard spots.

Digital rectal examination

The digital rectal examination (DRE) is an essential screening test for prostate disease, as well as for detecting other problems you may have in the lower rectum. However, the DRE also ranks among the least-desired parts of a physical exam because many men find it embarrassing or uncomfortable.

In fact, the test is quick and painless and takes place in the privacy of an examination room. You'll be asked to bend forward at the waist, with pants down, leaning against an exam table, or lie on your side on the table with your knees pulled up to your chest.

Your doctor first examines the outside of your anus for hemorrhoids or tiny breaks in the tissue (fissures). Then the doctor gently inserts a gloved finger, lubricated with gel, into your rectum.

Because the prostate gland is next to the rectum, your doctor can feel the back wall of the gland with his or her finger. By touching the gland, the doctor checks for bumps, irregularities, asymmetry, soft spots or hard spots in the prostate tissue that may suggest an abnormality.

A gland that feels enlarged may indicate benign prostatic hyperplasia (BPH). If the gland feels tender to the touch, it may be a sign of prostatitis. In addition, the outer portion of the gland is where 70 to 85 percent of cancerous tumors develop. In early stages of development, the tumors often feel like nodules or hard spots.

The DRE doesn't provide conclusive results — rather, it's an indicator of whether or not additional tests are required. For example, just because your doctor detects a hard spot on your prostate during a DRE doesn't mean you have cancer. Other conditions, including prostate infection or formation of small stones in the gland, can produce similar symptoms. The doctor will need other tests to help clarify the findings.

At the same time, just because the doctor doesn't feel any abnormalities doesn't mean there are no problems. A high percentage of prostate cancers, particularly in the early stages, are undetectable with a DRE.

Nevertheless, a Mayo Clinic study has found strong evidence that men who didn't receive regular DREs were more likely to die of prostate cancer than were a similar group of men who did have regular exams. The researchers believe that timely DREs could have saved the lives of 50 to 70 percent of these men.

Opinions differ among health care organizations as to when men should begin having DREs. Mayo Clinic urologists agree with the recommendation of the American Urological Association (AUA) that unless a man is at high risk, he should begin having annual DRE exams at age 50.

Urine test

As you may know, urine is fluid that transports waste products out of your body. The urine test detects various compounds in urine that may indicate a problem. A urine sample is collected, checked for color and appearance, and analyzed under a microscope.

- If your urine contains more white blood cells than is normal, you may have an infection in your prostate gland (prostatitis) or urinary tract.
- Red blood cells in your urine may signal inflammation of the prostate or, perhaps, a tumor. Other conditions, including bladder problems or inflammation of the urethra, also can produce blood in your urine.

- If your doctor thinks you have BPH, a urine test result that's normal can help confirm the diagnosis.

Prostate-specific antigen test

The doctor will take a blood sample from your arm and analyze it for a substance called prostate-specific antigen (PSA). The antigen is a compound produced in your prostate that helps liquefy semen — essential to the reproductive process. It's normal, however, for a small amount of PSA to circulate in your bloodstream.

PSA is a biological marker that can be used to detect disease. If higher-than-normal levels of PSA are measured in your blood, it could indicate prostate inflammation, enlargement or cancer. Most men have their first PSA test between the ages of 40 and 50.

Much as with the digital rectal exam (DRE), the PSA test is not conclusive evidence that you have an inflammation or cancer of the prostate — some men with high PSA counts end up having no problems with their prostates.

Rather, abnormal PSA test results indicate that you're at higher risk and that more tests may be necessary to help clarify what's causing the increase.

The PSA test is frequently used in conjunction with the DRE for initial prostate screening. However, many questions remain regarding how to interpret PSA test results and whether these findings should guide the course of prostate treatment. In a following section, beginning on page 29, the controversy surrounding PSA testing is discussed in greater detail.

Ultrasound

If there are concerns about the results of your digital rectal exam and PSA test, or following a general urinalysis or blood test, the doctor may want a more detailed look at your prostate gland. A procedure known as transrectal ultrasound can measure the size of your prostate and may indicate areas where cancer has developed.

Ultrasonography is an imaging technique that uses sound wave reflections to see inside your body. For an illustrated description of the procedure, see page 41. Because cancerous tissue is thicker and denser than healthy tissue, the sound wave reflections from a tumor may be different.

The procedure is harmless, although some men find it slightly uncomfortable. If the ultrasound images don't indicate that something is wrong, the doctor may feel that more tests are not needed. But if the ultrasound suggests the possibility of cancer, a biopsy will be needed to confirm its presence.

The PSA debate

The prostate-specific antigen (PSA) test was approved by the Food and Drug Administration in 1986 as a means to help detect prostate cancer. Since that time, the inclusion of this test in standard physical exams has been accompanied by a significant increase in the recorded number of cases of the disease. But controversy still remains over the dependability and utility of PSA test results.

The PSA test begins with a small amount of blood being drawn from a vein, usually from inside of your elbow. The sample is collected in an airtight vial and sent to a laboratory where a specialized procedure called an immunochemical assay determines how much PSA is circulating in your bloodstream.

A reading between 0 and 4 nanograms per milliliter (ng/mL) is considered normal. However, because PSA levels tend to naturally increase as you get older, some medical centers have adjusted their standards based on an individual's age (see "Mayo Clinic PSA standards" on page 30).

Just because your PSA level is above normal doesn't necessarily mean you have cancer. Some men have higher-than-normal PSA levels and healthy prostates. Other conditions in addition to cancer can increase the amount of PSA in your bloodstream.

Benign prostatic hyperplasia (BPH). Noncancerous enlargement of the prostate is the most common condition that can cause an elevated PSA reading. As prostate tissue grows, cells within the tissue produce more PSA — sometimes up to three times higher than normal.

Prostatitis. Irritation of the prostate gland due to inflammation or infection can cause cells to release or leak higher amounts of PSA into the bloodstream.

Cancer. Cancerous cells in the prostate may produce higher amounts of PSA than healthy cells do.

Mayo Clinic PSA standards

Mayo Clinic urologists use this age-adjusted scale to determine PSA normal upper limits,* based on the test used at Mayo.

Age	Upper limit ng/mL**	Age	Upper limit ng/mL	Age	Upper limit ng/mL	Age	Upper limit ng/mL
≤ 40	2.0	51	2.9	62	4.1	73	5.8
41	2.1	52	3.0	63	4.2	74	6.0
42	2.2	53	3.1	64	4.4	75	6.2
43	2.3	54	3.2	65	4.5	76	6.4
44	2.3	55	3.3	66	4.6	77	6.6
45	2.4	56	3.4	67	4.8	78	6.8
46	2.5	57	3.5	68	4.9	79	7.0
47	2.6	58	3.6	69	5.1	≥ 80	7.2
48	2.6	59	3.7	70	5.3		
49	2.7	60	3.8	71	5.4		
50	2.8	61	4.0	72	5.6		

*Upper limits increase almost every year as you age.

**Nanograms per milliliter

Factors other than disease may increase your PSA level. They include:

Ejaculation. The release of semen can cause a temporary increase in the PSA level in your blood. For that reason, some doctors have advised patients to abstain from sexual activity for up to two days before having their PSA exam. However, a study found that the increased levels of PSA after ejaculation dropped quickly and wouldn't likely result in abnormal test results. The researchers recommended that men not be asked to refrain from sexual activity before having the test.

Urinary tract infection. Similar to an infection in your prostate gland (prostatitis), a urinary tract infection can increase the PSA level in your blood.

Recent prostate treatment. Various procedures used to treat BPH — discussed in Chapter 5 — can temporarily irritate your prostate gland, producing abnormal levels of PSA. These procedures include:

- Prostate biopsy
- Transurethral resection of the prostate
- Transurethral incision of the prostate
- Prostate massage
- Microwave therapy of the prostate
- Laser therapy of the prostate

Following one of these procedures, wait from two weeks to two months before having a PSA test.

Concerns about accuracy

The PSA test detects prostate cancer in its early stages about 75 percent of the time. In about 25 percent of men with early prostate cancer, the results come back normal (less than 4 ng/mL). This is a major drawback of the test — if used as the only screening tool, the PSA test will not detect the early stages of prostate cancer in about one out of four men with the disease.

Another drawback of PSA testing is that the results don't distinguish between cancer and other prostate diseases. Among men with elevated PSA levels, only about one-third will have cancer. High PSA levels in the other two-thirds may be a result of BPH, prostatitis or other factors. As a result, many men who don't have cancer may nevertheless undergo testing that is expensive, time-consuming, and hard on their physical and emotional health.

Due to these drawbacks, not all doctors and medical organizations agree that the benefits of the PSA test outweigh its limitations. That's why this simple test remains controversial.

Benefits

Regular PSA screening can help identify prostate cancer long before any signs or symptoms become apparent. That's often when the cancer is still confined to the prostate gland. Localized cancer is much easier to treat and cure than cancer that has spread to other organs and tissues in the body.

Not all prostate cancers are alike. Some grow very slowly and remain within the prostate gland. Others are more aggressive and spread rather quickly to other organs. If your PSA test detects what turns out to be an aggressive form of prostate cancer, it could literally be a lifesaver.

The year 1995 marked the first-ever reduction in deaths from prostate cancer. Many doctors believe, and some studies support, that the PSA test was a major factor behind this decrease. However, health experts haven't been able to prove this link with certainty.

Limitations

The PSA test isn't completely reliable. In men in whom the test has failed to identify prostate cancer, it may give a false sense of security about their prostate health.

Among men with an elevated PSA, approximately two out of three may go through needless worry and unnecessary, expensive diagnostic procedures to learn that their condition is benign.

Whether the test leads to needless treatment is another question. If you have a slow-growing cancer, you may be able to monitor your condition and live with the cancer for years without it causing any problems.

Some men, however, find the waiting game difficult to accept. When they learn they have cancer, they want to do everything they can to get rid of it, opting for treatments such as surgery or radiation therapy. These treatments may produce strong side effects, including incontinence or impotence. This decreases the quality of life for men who might otherwise be living perfectly healthy, productive lives.

Finally, the issue of whether the early detection and treatment of prostate cancer actually saves lives remains unresolved. A Swedish study published in 2002 found that, in a group of men with the average age of 65, surgical treatment of early prostate cancer reduced prostate cancer deaths.

However, the same study found that after a six-year follow-up period, the mortality rates for all causes were fairly similar both in the group that had received treatment and the group that hadn't been treated.

BPH medications and PSA

Finasteride (Proscar) and dutasteride (Avodart) are medications commonly used to treat benign prostatic hyperplasia (BPH). They shrink the prostate gland by suppressing certain hormones that stimulate prostate growth. Finasteride is the same drug taken to promote hair growth in balding men and is sold under the brand name Propecia.

By altering hormone levels in the prostate gland, these drugs reduce production of PSA in the gland. The decrease in PSA is about 50 percent after 12 months of treatment and can occur even if you have prostate cancer, which would normally cause an increase in your PSA level.

This calls the accuracy of PSA testing into question for men who use these medications. Some doctors believe PSA tests aren't beneficial for men taking finasteride or dutasteride. Others, however, believe that the test can still be useful for tracking PSA ranges in men taking these medications — provided the ranges are adjusted. For example, if the normal PSA range for a 70-year-old man is 0 to 5.3 ng/mL, the normal range for a 70-year-old man taking finasteride or dutasteride might be 0 to 2.65 ng/mL.

It's essential for your doctor to be aware that you're taking these medications so that he or she can monitor and interpret the PSA results appropriately.

Possible answers?

Two large, long-term studies may provide some answers and help settle the PSA debate. However, it will be several years before the results are known.

PLCO. The Prostate, Lung, Colorectal and Ovarian Cancer Screening Trial is a large study sponsored by the National Cancer Institute to determine whether the methods of screening and the early detection of cancer save lives.

Screening methods for the prostate portion of the study are the DRE and PSA tests. Preliminary results indicate that about 14 percent of the men being screened showed suspicious results in their tests. Of those men, about 12 percent were diagnosed with prostate cancer within one year, most at an early stage. It's still too early to know how this knowledge impacts cancer deaths.

PIVOT. The Prostate Cancer Intervention Versus Observations Trial is funded by the Department of Veterans Affairs and the National Cancer Institute. The goal of PIVOT is to determine the best way to treat cancer that's confined to the prostate — whether to surgically remove the gland or let it alone and watch to see if the cancer spreads. Participants have regular checkups and respond to questionnaires regarding their quality of life.

Current recommendations

So, in the meantime, should you have a PSA test? There's still no definitive answer. Of the medical organizations that have taken a stand on the PSA test, about one-third support its use, one-third are neutral, and one-third don't support it.

The American Cancer Society (ACS), the National Comprehensive Cancer Network and the American Urological Association (AUA) are among its supporters. The ACS recommends the following schedules:

- Annual prostate checkup, including the PSA test and DRE, offered to all men over age 50
- Black men, because they're at higher risk, begin testing at age 45
- Men of any race with a family history of prostate cancer begin screening at age 40

As for how long you should continue testing, the ACS and AUA recommend lifelong screening. Many men in their 70s remain in excellent health and have good quality of life. They may have a life expectancy of at least 15 years and consequently would likely benefit from routine PSA testing.

Other organizations, however, suggest that after age 70 the test may no longer be necessary, particularly in cases where life expectancy is considered to be less than 10 years.

The American Medical Association (AMA) recommends that men be informed of the benefits and risks of prostate cancer screening, and that the

PSA test should be available to those who request it. The AMA has declined, however, to endorse mass screening for prostate cancer.

Mayo Clinic's view

Mayo Clinic specialists understand the pitfalls of the PSA test and agree that it's not perfect. But they support its use — in conjunction with the DRE — because it's the best screening tool available for detecting prostate cancer in its early stages.

Screening is especially beneficial for younger men who may have more curable cancers. As with many other cancers, the earlier prostate cancer is detected, the greater your chance for a complete recovery. Early detection also allows more time to consider all your treatment options.

In accordance with the ACS and the AUA, Mayo Clinic specialists recommend an annual PSA test beginning at age 50, unless you're at high risk of prostate cancer. If you're black or you have a family history of prostate cancer, you may want to begin at age 40.

If you have concerns about the PSA test — such as getting a false result or an abnormally high reading, or whether you're too old to have the test — discuss them with your doctor.

Improving PSA testing

Researchers continue looking for a more accurate screening method for prostate cancer that can reduce or eliminate some of the concerns regarding the current PSA procedure. Several options are being studied:

Free-PSA test. The PSA that circulates in your bloodstream comes in two forms — PSA that's bound to blood proteins and PSA that's unbound, or free PSA. The usual screening test measures both forms to determine the total amount of PSA in your blood.

Researchers have learned that making separate readings of bound and unbound PSA may help determine what kind of prostate problem you have. It turns out that there's higher levels of free PSA in your blood with benign conditions such as BPH. With prostate cancer, there's higher levels of bound PSA. The lower the percentage

Free-PSA test

The table below shows, based on your total PSA level, the probability of detecting cancer from a sample taken with needle biopsy.

Total PSA (ng/mL)	% Probability of cancer
0 to 2	about 1
2 to 4**	15
4 to 10	25

To further determine the probability of cancer when total PSA is in the 4 to 10 ng/mL range, your doctor may evaluate your free-PSA level. The higher the percentage of free PSA, the lower the probability of cancer.*

% Free PSA	% Probability of cancer
0 to 10	56
10 to 15	24
15 to 20	17
20 to 25	10
over 25	5

*Data are for men with normal digital rectal examination results, regardless of age.

**Normal PSA values may be less for younger men.

Adapted from the Journal of the American Medical Association, May 20, 1998

of free PSA on your test score, the more likely that cancer is responsible for the increase in your total PSA level. This would signal more testing, including prostate biopsy.

PSA velocity test. This test records the rate of change in your PSA levels over time. Although absolute totals can be key indicators, scientists also believe that the rate of change increases more rapidly in someone with prostate cancer than in someone with BPH or prostatitis. In other words, the faster that PSA levels climb over the course of several tests, the more likely that cancer has developed in your prostate.

PSA density test. This test compares your PSA level to the size of your prostate gland. What's known as prostate-specific antigen density (PSAD) is calculated by dividing your PSA level by your prostate volume.

An enlarged prostate (BPH) increases your PSA level, which can complicate a cancer diagnosis. A higher PSAD generally indicates a greater likelihood of prostate cancer. To get your prostate volume, your doctor would need to arrange a transrectal ultrasound.

The use of PSA density remains problematic because there's always the need for a second test, the ultrasound.

Ultrasensitive PSA test. This specialized test is capable of detecting minute quantities of PSA in your bloodstream. If you've already been treated for prostate cancer, the test may detect a recurrence of cancer far earlier than is possible with other tests — perhaps by one or two years.

Other markers

Other chemicals in the bloodstream may serve as markers for early-stage prostate cancer. They include:
- Human glandular kallikrein
- Chromogranin A
- Prostate-specific membrane antigen (PSMA)
- Early prostate cancer antigen 2 (EPCA-2)
- Prostate cancer gene 3 (PCA3)

Screening tests for these substances could eventually prove to be reliable indicators of prostate cancer.

New tests that measure the distribution of various proteins in the bloodstream — called serum proteomic patterns — may lead to more-accurate methods of determining whether high PSA levels actually mean prostate cancer. Such tests may be used instead of a biopsy to confirm the presence of disease.

Gene research. If researchers can identify a gene or genes responsible for prostate cancer, men who carry these genes could be monitored more closely to identify cancer in its very early stages. These men may even be able to prevent cancer through lifestyle changes, including a change of diet.

Answers to your questions

Can my family physician do a prostate examination?

Absolutely. Family physicians are vital to the process of screening men for prostate cancer or other abnormalities. The DRE and PSA tests are routine, and virtually every family doctor is familiar with them.

When should I see a urologist?

Your family doctor may recommend that you see a urologist if he or she has questions regarding your test results, suspects prostate cancer, or believes that a urologist could better treat non-cancerous conditions, such as BPH or prostatitis. If you have a problem urinating, your PSA level is elevated, or your family doctor finds an abnormality during a DRE, you may want to see a urologist.

Can I request a PSA test if my doctor routinely doesn't provide one?

Yes. Most health plans allow you to obtain the medical tests you desire.

However, the plan may not pay for the test. You may want to check with your doctor and your insurance provider to clarify whether a PSA test is covered by your insurance plan before requesting it. A PSA test costs less than $100.

My PSA level has always been very low. It's still within the normal range, but it has increased. Should I be concerned?

As you age, your PSA level may increase slightly. However, a noticeable change in your PSA should be followed with a thorough evaluation, even if the reading is normal.

Imaging techniques for the prostate

Being able to see inside the body is often necessary for a doctor to correctly diagnose and treat a prostate condition. Sophisticated imaging technology permits the doctor to study the structure and function of internal organs and identify abnormal conditions without the risk and discomfort of exploratory surgery.

In discussions with your doctor about prostate problems, you'll undoubtedly hear references to these imaging procedures — some of which you may be subjected to, including ultrasound, computerized tomography and magnetic resonance imaging. What do the different images show? How will the procedures help you? Are there any health risks or side effects?

This section may answer some of your questions and alleviate some of your concerns. The following pages describe the principle techniques and the images they produce. This information may help you better understand their importance in your health care.

Cystoscopy

A cystoscope is a thin tube made of flexible glass fibers, which can be inserted into your urethra and bladder. The tube is equipped with a small camera and light to display visuals on an external monitor — allowing your doctor to guide the device and see inside the structures. The scope can be manipulated in different directions by remote control.

The scope also contains open channels through which tiny instruments can be inserted to perform minor procedures, eliminating the need for open surgery — for example, removing tissue samples from the prostate or bladder (transurethral biopsy).

Cystoscopy is used to diagnose problems of the urinary tract and prostate, including polyps, tumors and abnormal growths, cancer, infection or inflammation, and causes of obstructed or painful urination.

When this device is used in other parts of the body, the procedure is called endoscopy. Cystoscopy is specific to an examination of the urinary tract.

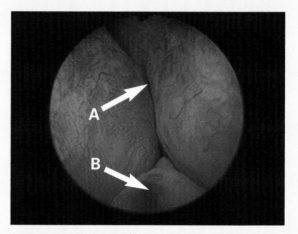

A cystographic image of the urethra at the apex of the prostate (arrow A). The ejaculatory duct is visible (arrow B), connecting the prostate and seminal vesicles for the production of sperm.

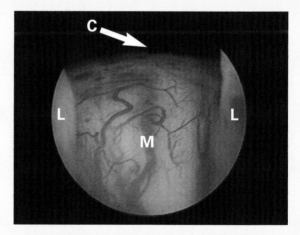

A cystographic image of the urethra at the bladder neck (arrow C). Two lateral lobes (L) and median lobe (M) of the prostate are visible.

Ultrasound

For the ultrasound procedure, a technician gently presses a small device (transducer) against your skin that emits high-frequency sound waves. Tissues and fluids inside your body — all of varying densities — reflect the sound waves back to the transducer. This device collects the echoes and relays them to a computer, which generates the image. The strength of an echo depends on the density of the tissue it's reflected from and how far away the tissue is.

Ultrasound images capture the function and movement of internal organs in real time, such as the narrowing of vessels and blockage of blood flow. Ultrasound can also guide doctors through delicate procedures such as a needle biopsy.

In a transrectal ultrasound, the transducer is attached to a probe and inserted into your rectum to get a better view of your prostate. The image can determine whether your prostate is enlarged and detect abnormal growths within the organ.

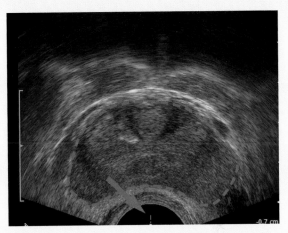

This axial transrectal ultrasound shows a normal prostate (red circle) with the urethra and the rectum (arrow).

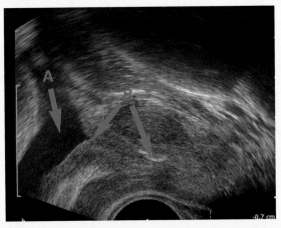

This sagital transrectal ultrasound shows a normal prostate with the bladder (arrow A) and urethra (arrow B).

X-ray

An X-ray machine emits a small burst of electromagnetic radiation through your body, which passes through bones, organs and soft tissue. Special film positioned on the other side of your body collects the signal, generating a 2-D image of your internal structures.

Different kinds of tissue absorb different amounts of the radiation. Dense tissue such as bone absorbs radiation well, so a weak signal reaches the film — bone appears as white on the film. Muscle and fat allow more radiation to pass than bone does, so they appear on X-ray film in different shades of gray. Hollow structures, such as the bowels, absorb little radiation — they appear dark on the film.

An X-ray can reveal the size and shape of internal organs such as the prostate. It can also indicate the location of a polyp, tumor or obstruction in the urethra. Sometimes, contrast dye will be added into your system to make hollow or fluid-filled structures such as the bladder or a blood vessel more visible on the X-ray.

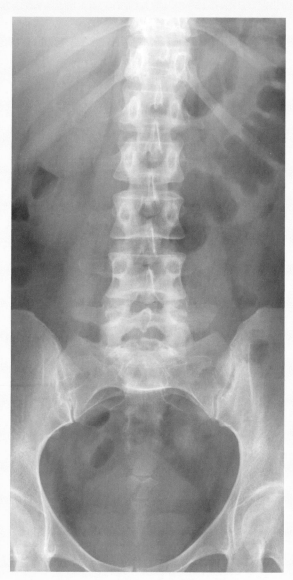

The image above is a standard X-ray of the abdomen and pelvic region. Dense tissue such as bone is the most prominently visible feature.

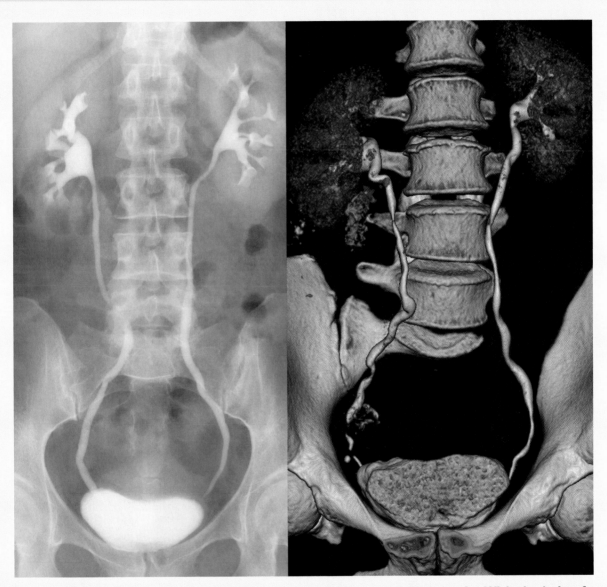

The left-hand image is an X-ray procedure known as excretory urography. With the help of contrast dye, a series of images taken at regular intervals reveals the kidneys, ureters and bladder — organs that may not show up well on a standard X-ray. In the right-hand image, special software has compiled the information into a volume-rendered, 3-D picture.

Computerized tomography

Computerized tomography (CT) combines X-rays with computers. The procedure makes multiple scans of your internal organs and tissue. Think of a loaf of bread that's been cut into slices — each CT scan represents a thin, cross-sectional slice of your body.

Standard X-rays are created by a stationary machine that focuses radiation on one part of your body. CT scans are created by a sophisticated X-ray unit that rotates around your body, emitting a series of narrow radiation beams. An X-ray detector rotates opposite this source, on the other side of your body, collecting the signals.

This procedure can detect hundreds of different levels of tissue density, in contrast to standard X-rays that detect only a few levels of density. A CT scan has a much greater degree of detail and clarity than standard X-rays do.

For the procedure, you'll lie on a table (gantry) that slides through a ring-shaped structure containing the X-ray unit. Small doses of radiation pass through your body at slightly different

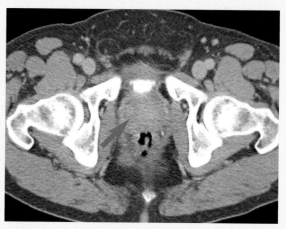

A CT image that shows a normal prostate (red arrow) and the pelvic region, taken in the axial plane. The hip bones are the large, white structures.

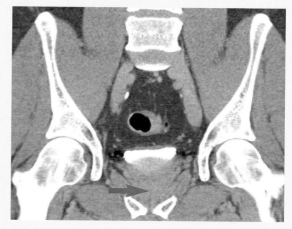

A CT image that shows a normal prostate (red arrow) and pelvic region taken in the coronal plane.

angles as the gantry slowly moves through the ring. A computer gathers the radiation signals. Each signal is interpreted on a scale ranging from black to white, according to the signal's intensity — similar to the creation of a standard X-ray.

A CT scan can locate stones, tumors, infections, obstructions and cancer. Also, doctors use this form of imaging to guide procedures such as biopsies and surgeries.

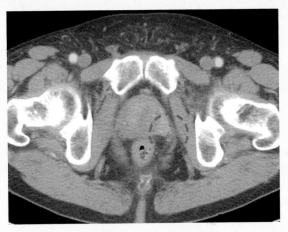

This axial CT image indicates the presence of cancer that has spread beyond the prostate — known as extraprostatic extension (red circle).

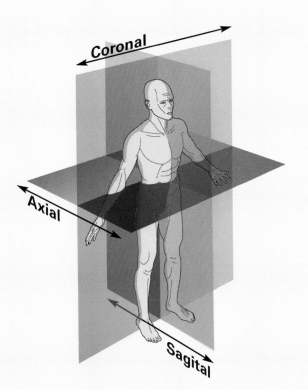

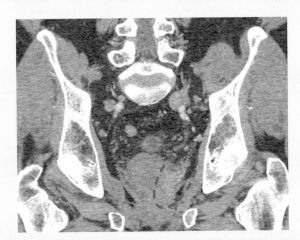

This CT image provides a coronal view of the same extraprostatic extension shown above (red circle).

Magnetic resonance imaging

Magnetic resonance imaging (MRI) creates cross-sectional pictures of internal organs, soft tissue and other structures, which can assist the doctor in diagnosing and treating prostate problems. MRI differs from computerized tomography (CT) because it uses a magnetic field and radio waves instead of radiation to create the image. MRI scans often provide much greater detail and clarity of soft tissue than CT scans do.

Typically, the MRI machine consists of a long cylindrical scanner equipped with strong magnets. As you lie on an examination table that slides through the cylinder, a magnetic field aligns all the atomic particles in your body. The aligned particles produce tiny signals that can be detected by a computer and made into images when the strong magnetic field is turned on and off.

MRI can be used to diagnose, treat and monitor a variety of conditions, including abnormalities of the urinary tract and reproductive tract, infection or enlargement of the prostate, and early detection of tumors and cancer.

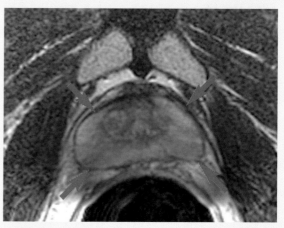

An axial MRI that shows a normal prostate with clearly defined borders (red arrows). The dark semicircle at the bottom of the image is the rectum.

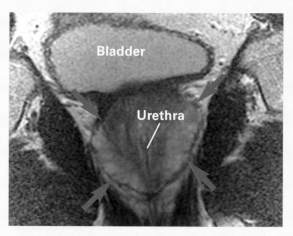

A coronal MRI that shows a normal prostate (red arrows) with the urethra at the center of the organ. The bladder lies directly above the prostate.

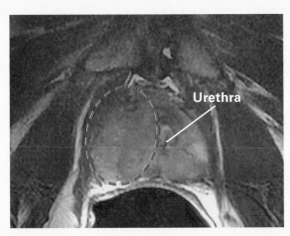

To the trained eye of a specialist, this axial MRI reveals a large tumor in the right lobe of the prostate (red circle), which has displaced the urethra to the left.

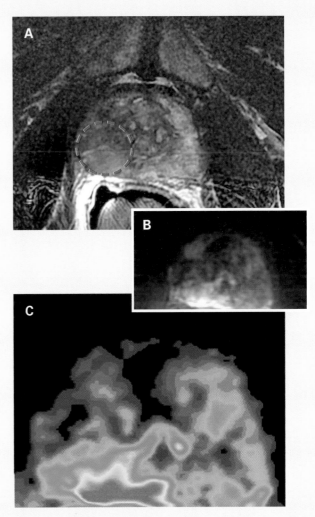

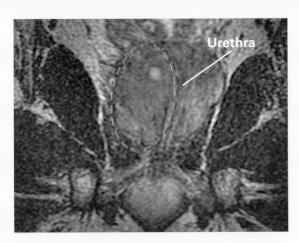

A coronal MRI of the prostate provides a different view of the tumor (red circle), which has spread outside the organ into surrounding tissue.

An axial MRI shows the location of a tumor in the right lobe (red circle in figure A). Contrast dye is used to create a dynamic contrast-enhanced (DCE) image (figure B). Color enhancement of the DCE provides a better definition of the tumor (red color in figure C).

Nuclear scan

Nuclear scanning — a subspecialty of radiology — introduces tiny amounts of radioactive materials called tracers (radionuclides) into your body to help visualize and evaluate medical conditions. The tracers travel through your bloodstream and accumulate in certain, designated tissues.

Wherever their location in your body, the tracers emit gamma-wave radiation, which is detected by a special camera that can generate images of the internal structures as well as biochemical processes taking place.

Different radionuclides are designed to go to different organs and tissues, so which tracer is selected for your test will depend on your symptoms. For example, one type of tracer collects in bone, while another goes to the kidneys. How much tracer is absorbed into the tissue may indicate the type of problem and how serious it is.

A nuclear scan provides different information than do an X-ray and ultrasound. The information is based on biological changes rather than structural ones. A radioactive tracer often detects disease at earlier stages than other diagnostic tests can — a critical factor in treating prostate cancer.

Nuclear scans can be superimposed over computerized tomography (CT) or magnetic resonance imaging (MRI) to correlate information from the different procedures. This process is known as image fusion.

The different kinds of nuclear imaging tests include bone scans, renal scans and positron emission tomography (PET). All of these procedures are important for diagnosing and treating prostate problems and some will be discussed on the following pages.

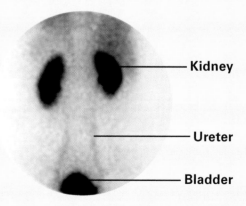

Renal scan showing kidneys and bladder.

Bone scan

A bone scan is a type of nuclear imaging in which the tracers injected into your body accumulate in your bones. Radiation emitted by these tracers is detected by a special camera. The scan reveals the metabolic state of your bones — the natural processes of bone growth, decay and renewal.

Specialists will study the scan looking for evidence of abnormal metabolism. Tracer material that accumulates in normal bone shows up in medium tones. Darker "hot spots" and lighter "cold spots" indicate where the tracer has or hasn't accumulated — often a sign of trouble.

Changes in metabolism can result from various problems, including tumors and joint infections. More importantly, a scan can reveal the presence of cancer, which may have spread, or metastasized from another location (red circles).

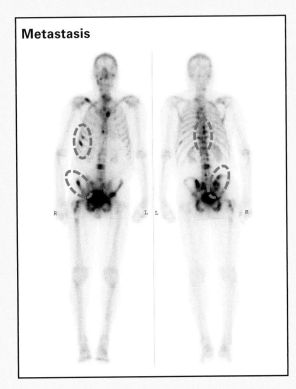

Normal

Metastasis

Positron emission tomography

Positron emission tomography (PET) is a form of nuclear imaging that measures the chemical processes taking place in your body. This can help doctors distinguish between the normal and abnormal function of different organs and tissues.

For the PET scan, you'll receive an injection of a tracer combined with glucose, choline or another substance, which your cells absorb and use for energy and metabolism. A special scanner detects the emission of this energy (positrons). The number of positrons detected indicates how much of the tracer was absorbed by the cells.

Cells that take up the most tracer are the most metabolically active — they appear on the scan as bright, intense colors, or "hot spots." Cells that don't take up as much tracer are less active (or they may have been damaged) — they appear as less intense colors, or "cold spots."

For example, cancerous tissue often uses more energy than surrounding tissue and appears as a hot spot on a PET scan. This helps your doctor determine the spread of cancer or assess how the cancer is responding to treatment. However, a PET scan must be interpreted carefully, and a biopsy is usually required to confirm the presence of cancer.

PET scans are often fused with computerized tomography (CT) or magnetic resonance imaging (MRI). In fact, many PET scanners are being produced with CT or MRI scanners already included.

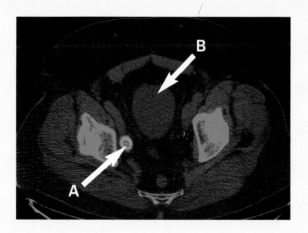

An axial image that fuses a PET scan with CT. It shows the bladder (B) and the presence of cancer, which has spread from the prostate to a nearby lymph node (A).

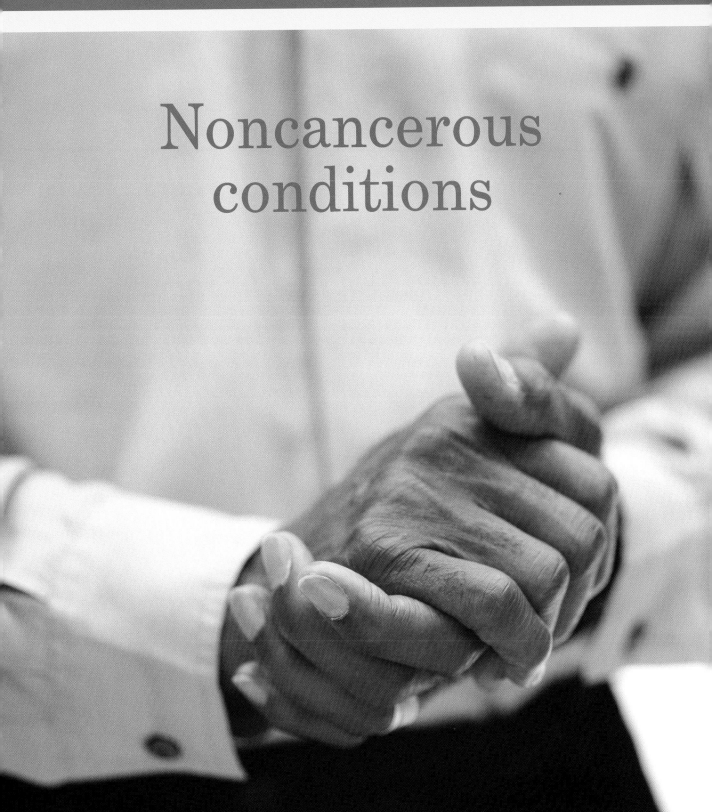

Part 2

Noncancerous conditions

Chapter 3

Prostatitis and chronic pelvic pain

One of the most common prostate problems men encounter is one you seldom hear about — unless you're a doctor. According to some estimates, up to a quarter of all visits men make to a doctor for genital or urinary problems are related to prostatitis and pain in the pelvic region.

Prostatitis is a general term for inflammation of the prostate gland. *Pelvic pain* refers to any pain, often nonspecific, in the area below your bellybutton and between your hips. Pelvic pain may be a symptom of another condition, or it can be classified as a condition in its own right.

If the pain lasts six months or longer, it's classified as chronic. There are many possible causes of chronic pelvic pain, including various disorders of the gastrointestinal, urinary or reproductive systems, and disruption of muscles or nerves. Diagnosing pelvic pain is a process of elimination until the most likely cause can be determined.

Chronic pelvic pain can frequently develop in men. Sometimes the symptoms are a result of persistent inflammation of the prostate gland. Other times, the pain is not related to the prostate at all and is spread throughout the pelvic region.

This chapter examines the four types of prostatitis, as well as common forms of chronic pelvic pain.

Types of prostatitis

Prostatitis is poorly understood and difficult to diagnose — in fact, many cases diagnosed as prostatitis end up having to do less with the prostate and more with the entire pelvic region.

Inflammation of the prostate may be due to an infection or another factor that's irritating the gland. The condition is not contagious and not a sexually transmitted disease.

The National Institutes of Health (NIH) has classified four distinct types of prostatitis (which are called categories):

- Category 1: acute bacterial prostatitis
- Category 2: chronic bacterial prostatitis
- Category 3: chronic pelvic pain syndrome — including the conditions previously known as nonbacterial prostatitis and prostatodynia
- Category 4: asymptomatic inflammatory prostatitis

The first three categories of prostatitis cause a variety of symptoms, including a frequent and urgent need to urinate and painful or burning sensations while urinating. This is often accompanied by pelvic, groin or low back pain. The fourth category of prostatitis has no symptoms. Identifying which category of prostatitis you have is crucial for treating the condition.

Unlike other prostate problems, you're more likely to develop prostatitis when you're younger, even before age 40. You're also at increased risk if you:

- Recently had an infection of the bladder or urethra
- Recently had a catheter inserted into your urethra
- Do not empty your bladder frequently enough and perform vigorous activities with a full bladder
- Jog or bicycle on a regular basis or ride horses

Men with HIV also are at increased risk of developing one of the bacterial forms of prostatitis.

Pain relievers and several weeks of treatment with an antibiotic are typically needed for categories 1 and 2 prostatitis. Adjunct therapy as well as self-care measures also may provide relief. Treatment for category 3 prostatitis is less certain and directed toward relieving symptoms. Category 4 prostatitis often doesn't require treatment.

Acute bacterial

The category 1 form of prostatitis is the least common but most evident form of the disease. A bacterial infection in the prostate gland produces a sudden, severe onset of signs and symptoms. These may include a combination of:

- Fever and chills
- Flu-like symptoms
- Pain in the lower back and genital area
- Urinary problems, including increased urgency and frequency, difficulty or pain when urinating, inability to completely empty the bladder, and blood-tinged urine
- Painful ejaculation

Bacteria normally found in the urinary tract or large intestine are most often responsible for this form of prostatitis. Most commonly, the acute infection starts in the prostate, but it can also spread from the bladder or urethra.

Acute bacterial prostatitis can lead to serious problems, including an inability to urinate and infection in the bloodstream (bacteremia). It's important to

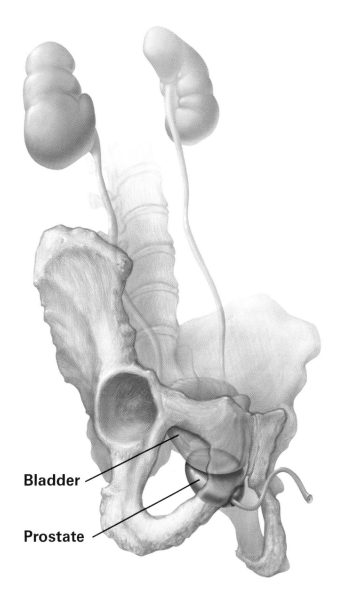

Bladder

Prostate

The urinary system and your prostate

The prostate gland is tucked into the pelvic region just below the bladder. Inflammation of the prostate may cause many urinary problems, as well as fever, chills and flu-like symptoms.

see your doctor immediately. Severe symptoms may require hospitalization for a few days until they improve.

Chronic bacterial

The category 2 form of prostatitis also is caused by a bacterial infection. Typically, chronic signs and symptoms develop gradually and they're often less severe than the acute form. They may include:

- Urinary problems, including increased urgency and frequency, difficulty starting or continuing urination, and diminished urine flow
- Pain or burning sensation when urinating
- Excessive nighttime urination
- Pain in the lower back and genital area
- Occasional blood in the semen (hematospermia)
- Painful ejaculation
- Slight fever
- Recurring bladder infection

What causes the chronic infection isn't clear. Sometimes it develops after an episode of acute prostatitis, when bacteria remain in the prostate. Other causes may include a bladder or blood infection, or after trauma to your urinary tract from activities such as bicycling or horseback riding.

Another way to cause a chronic infection in your prostate is with the insertion of an instrument or catheter into your urethra, which may carry bacteria with it. That's why some doctors prescribe antibiotics after the use of a urinary catheter.

Sometimes, stones form within the prostate tissue, serving as a location for recurring infection. On rare occasion, prostatitis results from an underlying structural or anatomical defect, which becomes a collection site for bacteria.

This form of prostatitis often becomes chronic because the infection has penetrated deep into the tissue. Even if antibiotics reach the bacteria, the infection may persist and cause symptoms.

Chronic pelvic pain syndrome

Most men with prostatitis have the category 3 form. Unfortunately, this form is also the most difficult to diagnose and treat. Instead of trying to eliminate the disease, the primary goals of treatment are often to relieve symptoms and improve quality of life.

When the NIH revised its classification system for prostatitis, it merged several

Prostatodynia

A condition merged into category 3 of the NIH prostatitis classification was called prostatodynia (pros-tuh-toe-DIN-ee-uh). Men would visit their doctors complaining of a dull pain "down there," meaning anywhere in the genital area.

Rather than being a problem with the prostate gland, prostatodynia may instead stem from the pelvic floor muscles. When you're under stress, you may not completely relax those muscles supporting your bladder and urethra, causing difficulties when you urinate. This theory could explain why most men with these symptoms tend to have Type A personalities — hard-driven, tense and stressed. Prostatodynia also seemed to occur frequently among marathon runners, bicyclists, triathletes, weightlifters and truck drivers.

conditions into category 3 that had previously been considered separate conditions, including chronic nonbacterial prostatitis and prostadynia (see sidebar above). This change was a recognition that often the symptoms involved more than just the prostate.

Chronic pelvic pain is a syndrome — a collection of signs and symptoms that occur in a recognizable sequence or pattern. In diagnosing the condition, a doctor will need to evaluate many factors, including the location of pain and discomfort, severity of the symptoms, problems with urination, and impact on quality of life.

In fact, the signs and symptoms of chronic pelvic pain syndrome are very similar to those for chronic bacterial prostatitis — both in kind and in severity — although it's unlikely that you'll develop a fever.

The doctor may try to distinguish this syndrome from a bacterial form of prostatitis by studying lab tests to find out

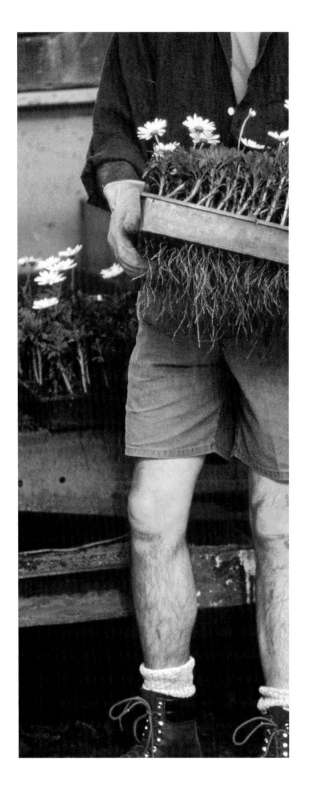

whether bacteria is present in your urine or prostate gland fluid. With chronic pelvic pain syndrome, the doctor will not find bacteria in the sample but on occasion may detect white blood cells — a sign of inflammation within the prostate.

The primary reason why chronic pelvic pain syndrome is so difficult to treat is because the cause is so uncertain. Theories abound as to possible triggers. However, no factors are definite and many aren't well understood. Among the possible causes are:

Heavy lifting. Lifting heavy objects while your bladder is full may cause urine to back up and seep into your prostate, causing inflammation.

Sexual activity. Sexually active young men who have an inflammation of the urethra (urethritis) or sexually transmitted disease, such as gonorrhea or chlamydia, are more likely to develop the syndrome. In some men, having less sexual intercourse also may be a contributing factor.

Anxiety or stress. These may cause you to tighten the urinary sphincter muscle — which controls urine flow from the bladder — and the muscles supporting the bladder and rectum (pelvic floor muscles). This prevents the muscles from relaxing, which may irritate your prostate or cause fluids in the urethra to back up into the prostate.

Pelvic muscle spasm. Urinating in an uncoordinated manner when the internal sphincter muscle isn't relaxed may lead to high pressure and inflammation in the prostate.

Other infectious agents. The inflammation may be caused by a nonbacterial infectious agent that standard laboratory tests haven't detected.

Occupational factors. This form of prostatitis is associated with certain occupations that subject the prostate to a great deal of vibration, such as truck driving or operating heavy machinery.

Physical activities. Frequent participation in activities such as bicycling or jogging may irritate the prostate gland.

Whatever the initial trigger, the combination of inflammation and nerve irritation can result in chronic nerve sensitization — a process in which pain messages being sent to the brain are too severe and out of proportion to the circumstances.

Sensitization may affect entire neurological pathways, including the sensing, feeling and thinking centers of your brain. Once nerve activation of this kind is established, many factors can stimulate the sensitized pathways and cause frequent symptom flare-ups — for example, excessive amounts of caffeine or high levels of stress may bring on the condition.

Asymptomatic inflammatory

Inflammation can occur in the prostate without producing any symptoms — which is why the name for this category 4 form of prostatitis includes the word *asymptomatic.* Typically, the condition is discovered indirectly — for example, during a biopsy to check the prostate tissue for cancer.

The cause of asymptomatic inflammation in the prostate is unknown. As well, little is known about its long-term effects and there's no effective means of treating it. While asymptomatic inflammatory prostatitis is not cancerous, there's some speculation that it could be a precursor to prostate cancer. More research is needed to understand this mysterious condition.

Diagnosis

Most men have a prostate checkup in conjunction with their regular physical exams. If your doctor doesn't perform a digital rectal exam when you have this routine physical, ask whether you should have one.

See your doctor if you develop any of the signs and symptoms of prostatitis, such as persistent urinary discomfort and pain, blood-tinged urine or semen, or pain while ejaculating — especially if these symptoms come on suddenly. When left untreated, prostatitis can lead to more serious problems, for example, the infection could spread to other parts of your body.

Two important steps in diagnosing prostatitis are (1) ruling out any other condition that may be causing the symptoms and (2) determining the type of prostatitis you have.

To start, your doctor will ask you questions about your symptoms: What are they? Do they come and go, or are they persistent? When did they first occur? Can you recall any changes in your lifestyle that took place about the time the symptoms began?

Your doctor may also ask you about recent medical procedures that you've had, as well as previous infections, your sexual habits, your occupation, and whether you have a family history of prostate problems.

Often, a urine sample is collected at the beginning of the exam to check for evidence of urinary tract infection.

The physical examination generally includes checking your abdomen and pelvic area for unusual tenderness. During a digital rectal examination (DRE), your doctor manually examines your prostate gland by gently inserting a lubricated, gloved finger into your rectum (see pages 26-27). An inflamed prostate often feels enlarged and tender to the touch.

Prostate fluid can be collected for evaluation by rubbing rather vigorously against the gland with the gloved finger, forcing the fluid into your urethra where it combines with urine and exits through the penis. This procedure is often referred to as prostate massage or prostate stripping.

A urine sample is taken at this point that includes fluid from the prostate massage. This fluid is examined under a microscope for evidence of bacteria and white blood cells. The presence of bacteria points to an infection. White blood cells indicate inflammation.

If your urine tests positive for both inflammation and infection, you likely have bacterial prostatitis and can be treated with antibiotics.

If the sample includes white blood cells but no bacteria, you probably have a form of chronic pelvic pain syndrome and can be treated for symptom relief.

If neither bacteria nor white blood cells are found in the urine sample, your symptoms may be related to other disorders, requiring more tests.

For men with a higher risk of prostate cancer, the doctor may order PSA testing. Tests may also be taken to measure urine flow rate and residual volume after urination, to check for benign prostatic hyperplasia (BPH).

For other men, the doctor may recommend further evaluation with X-rays, ultrasound, cystoscopy and specialized studies of bladder function. These tests may reveal tumors, bladder or urethral dysfunction, and other kidney or bladder problems.

Treatment

Once your doctor has identified the category of prostatitis you have, you can work together on developing a plan to treat the condition and, for the bacterial forms, possibly cure it.

Since the cause of chronic pelvic pain syndrome (category 3) is often unknown, treating this form of prostatitis is difficult. However, with some patience and experimentation, many men find ways to manage the condition and keep it from interfering seriously with their daily lives.

Medications

One or more of the following drugs may help eliminate or control your symptoms. Often, these medications are more effective at the beginning — early in the course of the drug — but become less effective over time.

Antibiotics. Antibiotics are a traditional first line of treatment for all forms of prostatitis. Your doctor will likely start you on a drug that fights a broad spectrum of bacteria. If the specific type of bacterium that's causing your infection can be identified — based on urine and

Prostatitis symptom index

Record answers to the following questions that best describe your symptoms. Discuss your answers with your health care provider.

Pain or discomfort

1. In the last week, have you had any pain or discomfort in the following areas?
    a. Area between the rectum and the testicles (perineum)
    b. Testicles
    c. Tip of the penis (not related to urination)
    d. Below your waist, in your pubic or bladder area

2. In the last week, have you experienced:
    a. Pain or burning during urination?
    b. Pain or discomfort during or after sexual climax?

3. How often have you had pain or discomfort in any of these areas over the last week?
    0 Never   1 Rarely   2 Sometimes   3 Often   4 Usually   5 Always

4. Which number best describes your average pain or discomfort on the days that you had it over the last week?
    1   2   3   4   5   6   7   8   9   10
    No pain   Extremely severe pain

Urination

5. How often have you had a sensation of not emptying your bladder completely after you finished urinating during the last week?
    0 Not at all
    1 Less than one in five times
    2 Less than half the time
    3 About half the time
    4 More than half the time
    5 Almost always

6. In the last week, how often have you had to urinate again fewer than two hours after you finished urinating?

    0 Not at all
    1 Less than one in five times
    2 Less than half the time
    3 About half the time
    4 More than half the time
    5 Almost always

Impact of symptoms

7. In the last week, have your symptoms kept you from your usual activities?

    0 None
    1 Only a little
    2 Some
    3 A lot

8. How much did you think about your symptoms during the last week?

    0 None
    1 Only a little
    2 Some
    3 A lot

Quality of life

9. If you were to spend the rest of your life with your symptoms just the way they have been during the last week, how would you feel about that?

    0 Delighted
    1 Pleased
    2 Mostly satisfied
    3 Mixed (about equally satisfied and dissatisfied)
    4 Mostly dissatisfied
    5 Unhappy
    6 Terrible

Adapted from National Institutes of Health, Chronic Prostatitis Symptom Index, 2008

prostate fluid samples — a different drug may be prescribed that's more effective at killing the bacteria.

How long you'll take an antibiotic will depend on how well you respond to the drug. If you have acute bacterial prostatitis, you may need medication for a few weeks — you may also need to be hospitalized in order to receive the antibiotics intravenously.

Chronic bacterial prostatitis, on the other hand, is often more resistant to antibiotics, making the drugs less effective. It takes longer to cure the infection — often six to 12 weeks — and sometimes the infection may never be eliminated. In addition, you may have a relapse as soon as you stop taking the drug. This would require a daily low-dose antibiotic for an indefinite period to keep the infection under control.

Even though chronic pelvic pain syndrome isn't caused by bacterial infection, some doctors will prescribe an antibiotic for a few weeks to see if it improves symptoms. For unknown reasons, some men with this condition seem to benefit from a continuous low dose of an antibiotic. If the drug doesn't help, your doctor will recommend that you stop taking it.

Alpha blockers. If you're having difficulty urinating, perhaps due to an obstruction in your urinary tract, your doctor may prescribe an alpha blocker. Alpha blockers help relax the bladder neck and the muscle fibers where the prostate adjoins the bladder. This can improve urine flow and help empty your bladder more completely.

Alpha blockers may also decrease the backflow of urine into the prostate, which may help control prostatitis.

Pain relievers. Over-the-counter pain relievers, such as aspirin, ibuprofen (Motrin, Advil, others) and acetaminophen (Tylenol, others), can help relieve pain and discomfort. They may also help break the pain cycle brought on by sensitized nerves.

Keep in mind that taking too much of any of these medications can cause serious side effects including abdominal pain and intestinal bleeding. Check first with your doctor before taking any pain reliever.

Muscle relaxants. Spasms of the pelvic muscles may accompany prostatitis. On rare occasion, combining muscle relaxant medication with other medications to treat prostatitis may be helpful.

Lifestyle changes

For reasons that are unclear, some men with chronic prostatitis find that making simple lifestyle changes such as avoiding long periods of sitting or not eating certain foods and beverages seems to improve their condition. Some of the more common practices include:

- Drinking plenty of water
- Limiting alcohol, caffeine and highly spiced foods
- Going to the bathroom at regular intervals
- Having regular sexual activity
- If you're a bicyclist, using a "split" bicycle seat that reduces pressure on the prostate

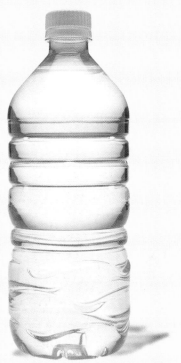

Although these practices don't appear to cause any harm, studies have yet to show that changes in dietary, bathroom or sexual habits can actually cure prostatitis or relieve its symptoms.

That doesn't mean that if you find such practices helpful you should discontinue them. Living with chronic prostatitis often comes down to limiting some things that seem to make the condition worse and doing other things that seem to improve it — without knowing why or how the changes help.

If you have prostatitis, you may experiment with various lifestyle changes, but do so gradually and always inform your doctor of your intentions.

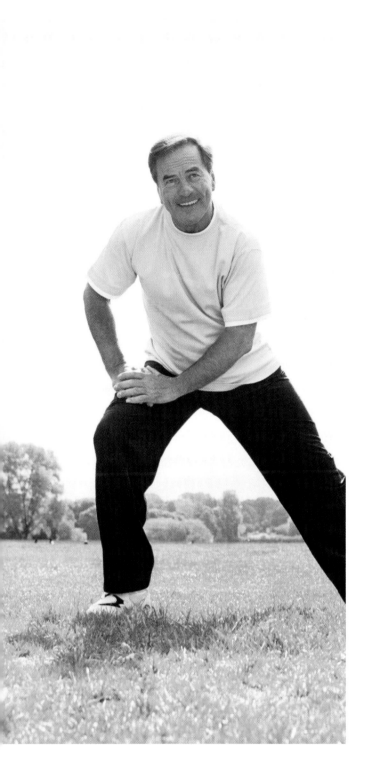

Physical therapy

Special exercises and relaxation techniques can improve the symptoms of prostatitis in some men, perhaps because tight or irritated muscles may be contributing to prostatitis. Common techniques include:

Exercise. Stretching and relaxing the lower pelvic muscles may help relieve your symptoms. Sometimes, the addition of heat with a low electric current — known as diathermy — may make the muscles more limber.

A physical therapist can show you which exercises will benefit you the most and how to perform them. You can then regularly do the exercises yourself at home.

Biofeedback. This technique teaches you how to control body responses to certain stimuli. A trained therapist can help you get started — but you learn how to produce the changes yourself, such as slowing your heart rate or relaxing your muscles.

Sitz bath. From the German word *sitzen*, meaning "to sit," this type of bath simply involves sitting and soaking the lower half of your body in warm water. Many men find this therapy relieves pain and relaxes the lower abdominal muscles. Few treatments are easier or as relaxing to do.

When your condition is first diagnosed, the doctor may recommend taking sitz baths two or three times a day for 30 minutes each time. For acute bacterial prostatitis, keep the water temperature below 99 F. If you have chronic prostatitis, temperatures up to 115 F are fine.

Surgery

Surgical removal of the infected portion of the prostate may be an option in a few severe cases when other treatments haven't work. However, the chance of having a positive outcome from major surgery for any type of prostatitis is quite low. For this reason, most doctors are hesitant to perform surgery for prostatitis, and generally discourage the procedure, even as a last resort.

Herbal therapy

The claims that certain natural remedies are helpful for prostatitis are unsubstantiated and await rigorous scientific study. Nevertheless, some men report that products such as saw palmetto, bee pollen extract, zinc supplements and quercetin have helped them manage their symptoms.

Keep in mind, a product's claim to being "natural" doesn't always translate into being safe. The supplement industry is unregulated, and few well controlled studies have been undertaken to determine efficacy or possible interactions. Always consult your doctor before using any supplement.

Answers to your questions

Does prostatitis increase my risk of cancer?

There's no evidence that acute or chronic prostatitis puts you at greater risk of prostate cancer. Prostatitis may, however, increase the level of prostate-specific antigen (PSA) in your blood. If your PSA level is elevated and you have prostatitis, it's advisable to redo the test after you've been treated with antibiotics. If you have chronic prostatitis, your doctor may test your free-PSA level (see "Free-PSA test" on pages 35-36).

Can I pass on a prostate infection to my partner during intercourse?

Prostatitis can result from a sexually transmitted disease, but prostatitis itself isn't contagious. Prostatitis can't be passed on through sexual intercourse, so your partner doesn't have to worry about catching an infection.

Can prostatitis make me infertile?

It may. The disease can interfere with the development of semen, making it difficult for the fluid to ejaculate properly during intercourse. Because semen carries sperm, this may lower your fertility rate. A few studies indicate the presence of poor sperm quality in some men with prostatitis.

Is surgery ever used to treat the disease?

Generally, doctors prefer nonsurgical procedures. But if the disease has drastically affected your fertility, antibiotics aren't able to improve your symptoms, or you're unable to urinate, your doctor might recommend surgery. A surgeon may try to open blocked ducts in the gland to relieve congestion and help semen flow more freely. Surgery isn't recommended for chronic nonbacterial disease.

Can the herb saw palmetto help relieve my symptoms?

Studies show that saw palmetto is not as effective a treatment for noncancerous enlargement of the prostate gland (benign prostatic hyperplasia) as once thought. Furthermore, there's no evidence that this popular herb relieves infection or inflammation associated with prostatitis. Saw palmetto is discussed later on pages 233-234.

Chapter 4

Understanding benign prostatic hyperplasia

At birth, your prostate gland is about the size of a pea. It grows slightly during childhood, and then at puberty — your early teen years — it typically undergoes rapid growth. By the time you reach age 20, your prostate is fully developed.

Most men, however, experience a second period of prostate growth. In their mid-40s, cells near the center of the prostate gland — in the transitional zone that surrounds the urethra — begin to grow more rapidly than normal. As tissue in this zone enlarges, it often presses on the urethra and obstructs urine flow. *Benign prostatic hyperplasia* is the medical term for this condition. It's commonly called BPH.

Having BPH does not put you at higher risk of prostate cancer. Although abnormal tissue growth is associated with both conditions, the growths occur very differently. Prostate cancer develops in the outer sections of the gland, often spreading outward into surrounding tissue. BPH develops in the gland's interior and grows inward, constricting the urethra. Although some symptoms of BPH mimic those of cancer, it's a benign condition.

A fact of life

The chance that you'll develop BPH increases with age, particularly after age 40. That's when your prostate — primarily in the transitional zone — begins the second growth spurt. BPH affects more than half of men in their 60s and about 90 percent of men in their 80s.

As the growth takes place, prostate tissue becomes lumpy, forming the characteristically uneven clusters of cell masses. Smooth muscle in the prostate reacts to this buildup by constricting and tightening around the urethra, narrowing the channel. This obstructs urine flow from the bladder.

The cause or causes of this prostate enlargement is unknown. Researchers believe that as you age, your prostate becomes more susceptible to the effects of male hormones, including testosterone. These hormones make certain cells in the prostate grow.

Other factors likely play a role in the development of BPH. Family history can increase your odds of developing the disease, pointing to a possible genetic link. BPH is more common in Caucasian men than in men of Asian descent, which may also suggest a lifestyle component. For unknown reasons, married men are more likely to get BPH than are single men.

Signs and symptoms

The signs and symptoms of BPH can be extremely disruptive for some men, and pose few problems for others. The impact varies according to the size and shape of new tissue growth, the location of the growth inside your prostate, and its effect on your bladder.

Only about half the men who develop BPH experience signs and symptoms that are noticeable or annoying enough for them to seek medical treatment. These signs and symptoms may include:

- Frequent urination, including repeated awakening at night to urinate (nocturia)
- Weak urine stream (flow rate)
- Difficulty starting urination, or alternately starting and stopping during urination
- Extended period of dribbling at the end of urination
- Sudden urgency to urinate, sometimes leading to involuntary leakage
- Feeling that the bladder is full or not being able to empty the bladder

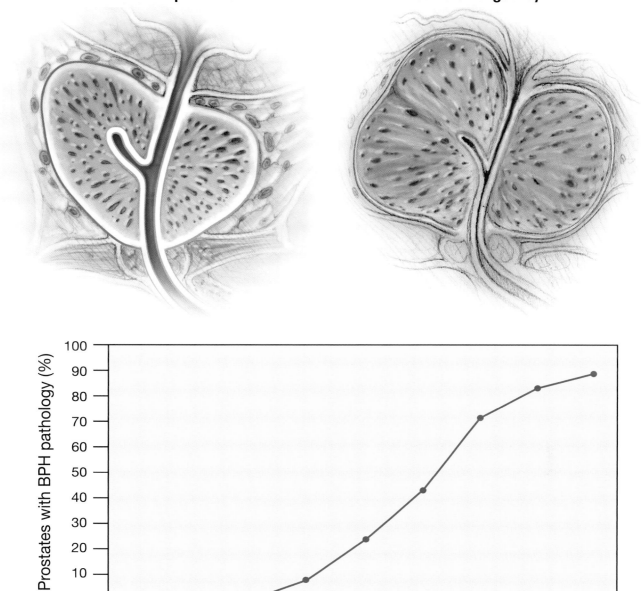

Normal prostate

Prostate enlarged by BPH

BPH prevalence

The increasing prevalence of BPH with age does not mean signs and symptoms developed in every case. Data was collected from microscopic examinations of prostates at autopsy.

At first, BPH may cause few symptoms because the strong bladder muscle can still force urine through the narrowed urethra. But these strong contractions also cause the bladder wall to thicken and become less elastic — which only makes you want to urinate more often and with greater urgency.

You may start avoiding social events so that you won't face long lines to the bathroom. You may be waking up tired in the morning from frequent night-time trips to empty your bladder. You may no longer wear light-colored pants for fear of noticeable dribbling.

A larger prostate doesn't always mean you'll have more severe symptoms — it just depends on how much the internal growth of tissue has affected the urethra and bladder.

Furthermore, signs and symptoms of BPH don't necessarily get worse over time. According to one survey, mild to moderate symptoms worsened about 20 percent of the time, improved in another 20 percent, and stayed about the same for the rest of the group.

For some men, the bladder becomes small and muscular and can no longer hold as much as it used to. For other men, the bladder becomes stretched out, loses muscle tone and never drains completely. When you can't completely empty your bladder, BPH becomes a serious health threat, with recurrent bladder infection and kidney damage, which may be accompanied by fever, vomiting and back pain.

Getting a diagnosis

If you're experiencing urinary problems, describe the symptoms at your next medical visit. Your doctor can determine whether you have BPH and if your symptoms require treatment.

If you don't find your symptoms annoying and they don't pose a health threat, treatment may not be necessary. But that doesn't mean it's all right to let urinary symptoms go unchecked.

Instead of BPH, your symptoms could be early warning of a more serious condition, including bladder stone, bladder infection, bladder cancer, side effects of medication, heart failure, diabetes, a neurological problem, prostatitis or prostate cancer.

To better understand your condition, your doctor will ask you questions about the symptoms, when they developed, and how often they occur. The doctor will also ask about other health problems you may have, medications you may be taking, and whether there's a history of prostate problems in your family.

In addition, your checkup may include:

- A digital rectal examination to see whether your prostate is enlarged and to help rule out prostate cancer
- A urine test to rule out an infection or a condition that can produce similar symptoms
- A prostate-specific antigen (PSA) blood test to help rule out cancer

If the results of these tests suggest BPH, your doctor may want to perform additional exams. These new tests help confirm the diagnosis of BPH and determine its severity.

Prostate symptom index

The American Urological Association (AUA) developed a series of questions regarding specific symptoms associated with BPH. As part of an exam, you rank how severely each symptom affects you on a scale of 1 to 5.

The index score, which is the sum of your rankings, helps measure how severely these symptoms affect your daily life (see pages 74-75).

What's known as your International Prostate Symptom Score (IPSS) adds a specific quality-of-life question to the AUA index. This additional question is based more on personal feeling — it helps gauge how bothered you are by your symptoms.

The question considers spending the rest of your life with the symptoms just as they are. Only you can respond honestly about how you would feel. Your answer, called your bother score, is based on a scale from 0 to 6, with 0 being delighted and 6 being terrible. The bother score may help decide what, if any, treatment is appropriate.

For example, someone who has moderate symptoms according to the AUA rankings but a low bother score may be happier with no or minimally invasive treatment rather than risking the potential side effects of a more invasive procedure. On the other hand, someone with the same symptoms and a high bother score may be willing to tolerate side effects of a more invasive treatment in order to get relief.

Prostate symptom index

The American Urological Association symptom index for benign prostatic hyperplasia (BPH) is designed to help doctors evaluate BPH severity.

Symptom description

Over the past month, how often have you had a *sensation of not emptying* your bladder completely after you finished urinating?

Over the past month, how often have you had to *urinate again less than two hours* after you had finished urinating?

Over the past month, how often have you found you *stopped and started* again several times when you urinated?

Over the past month, how often have you found it is *difficult to postpone urination*?

Over the past month, how often have you had a *weak urinary stream*?

Over the past month, how often have you had to *push or strain* to begin urination?

Over the past month, how many times did you most typically *get up to urinate* from the time you went to bed *at night* until you got up in the morning?

Scoring key
Mild symptoms: 1 to 7 total points
Moderate symptoms: 8 to 19 total points
Severe symptoms: 20 to 35 total points

Quality of life (bother score)
If you were to spend the rest of your life with these symptoms just the way they are, how would you feel about that?

Adapted from American Urological Association Education and Research, 2003

Not at all	Less than 1 time in 5	Less than half the time	Almost half the time	More than half the time	Almost always	Score
0	1	2	3	4	5	_____
0	1	2	3	4	5	_____
0	1	2	3	4	5	_____
0	1	2	3	4	5	_____
0	1	2	3	4	5	_____
0	1	2	3	4	5	_____
None 0	**1 time** 1	**2 times** 2	**3 times** 3	**4 times** 4	**5 or more times** 5	_____

Total score _____

Delighted	**Pleased**	**Mostly satisfied**	**Mixed**	**Mostly dissatisfied**	**Unhappy**	**Terrible**
0	1	2	3	4	5	6

Your responses to the prostate symptom index may influence the process to determine your best treatment (see the diagnostic tree on page 77). If you and your doctor believe your symptoms have become too bothersome, other tests may be considered to assess your condition and determine if more invasive treatment is necessary.

Urodynamic studies

If there's suspicion that your symptoms are related more to the bladder than to the prostate, a series of tests can help your doctor assess bladder function — how much urine it can hold, how much pressure builds up inside, and how full it gets when you feel the urge to urinate. Collectively, these are known as urodynamic studies.

Urinary flow test. This test measures the volume of urine that you expel from your bladder per second. The results may suggest an obstruction in your urinary tract or a problem with your pelvic muscles. Keep in mind that flow rate normally decreases as you age.

You'll urinate into a special machine in the privacy of a testing room. A flow rate of more than 15 milliliters per second (mL/s) is normal or signifies only mild disease. A rate of 10 to 15 mL/s is often associated with moderate symptoms, and less than 10 mL/s usually indicates severe BPH.

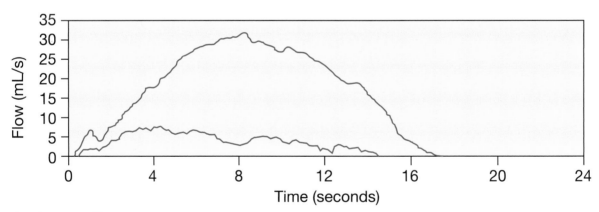

Urinary flow test

The red line on this graph indicates a normal urinary flow rate, with a peak of around 30 mL/s and an average rate of approximately 20 mL/s. The blue line is a low flow rate that may indicate someone with severe BPH.

Postvoid residual test. After you finish urinating (postvoid), some urine may remain in your bladder (residual) — the amount may vary each time you urinate. Retaining too much urine can cause problems. Urine backup is often a breeding ground for bacteria, leading to recurrent urinary tract infections and kidney damage.

This test determines how well you can empty your bladder and, if not, measures how much urine you retain. If you retain more than about 100 milliliters (about a half cup) in your bladder, you may need further evaluation.

There are two ways to perform this test — either by inserting a flexible catheter into your bladder or by using ultrasound imaging. Ultrasound is a more common method but provides a less accurate reading.

Cystometry. A small catheter is threaded into your bladder containing a pressure-measuring device called a cystometer. Water is slowly injected into your empty bladder until you feel the need to urinate.

A pressure flow study compares the pressure inside your bladder to the force of urine leaving your penis. It

will also measure the activity of the pelvic floor muscles that keep urine from leaking. This test helps identify obstruction that can occur from BPH.

Cystoscopy

In this procedure, a flexible instrument equipped with a lens and light system (cystoscope) is inserted through your urethra. It allows your doctor to see inside the urethra — including the part surrounded by the prostate — and the inside of the bladder. The procedure can detect prostate enlargement, obstruction of the urethra or bladder neck, an anatomic abnormality, or the

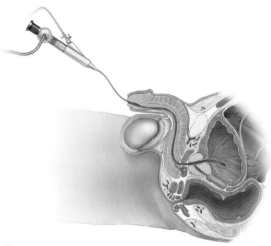

Cystoscopy

A narrow, flexible tube inserted through the penis and urethra allows the doctor to examine the inside of your bladder.

development of stones in your bladder. For more information on cystoscopy, see page 40. Other imaging tests may be used, including ultrasound and computerized tomography (CT).

Intravenous pyelogram

An intravenous pyelogram (PI-uh-lo-gram) is an X-ray procedure that helps detect urinary obstructions. For the procedure, a contrast dye is injected into a vein and collects in the kidneys. X-ray images with the dye reveal any abnormalities in the urinary tract as it passes through the system.

The development of newer and more detailed imaging techniques, such as CT, has led to less frequent use of the intravenous pyelogram procedure.

Next steps

The decision tree on page 79 is a visual guide that may help you navigate a pathway through common diagnosis and treatment options for BPH. This guide is a general one — and your experience may differ according to your signs and symptoms, age, physical health and doctor's recommendations.

The path that these decisions will take is influenced strongly by how well you tolerate lower urinary tract symptoms, if you're experiencing them — your IPSS "bother" score (see pages 73-76). Each person's tolerance capacity may vary considerably from what others can deal with. You and your doctor must determine your comfort range, and when you know that you've exceeded it.

The location of the AUA/IPSS symptom index in the decision-tree schema immediately follows the initial evaluation by your doctor. Mild symptoms of BPH (an AUA/IPSS score of 7 or less) may result in nothing more than careful monitoring. Moderate to severe symptoms (a score of 8 or more) usually require more tests and treatment.

Decades ago, the only treatment for BPH was surgery. If you had the condition, you would wait until the symptoms were severe enough to consider surgical removal of obstructing prostate tissue.

More recently, other treatment options have become available, including medications and less invasive therapies. These are often the first choice of treatment, although many men will eventually require surgery. Your options are discussed in greater detail in Chapter 5.

BPH decision tree

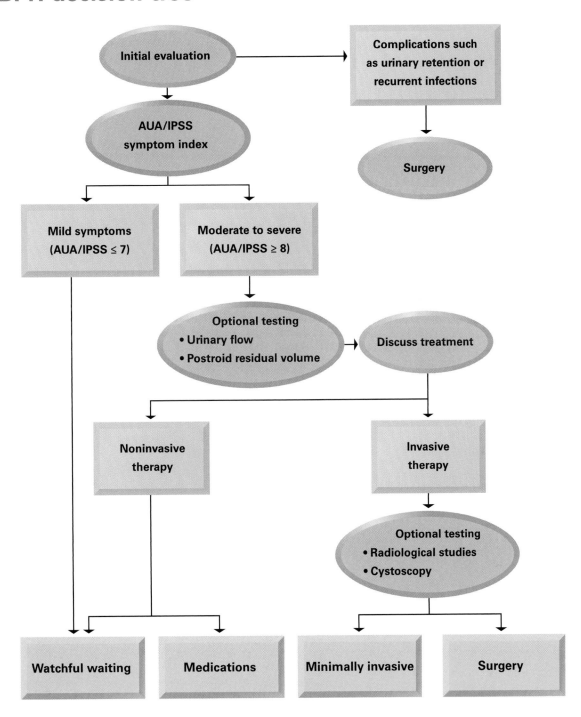

Answers to your questions

Are the tests used to diagnose BPH painful?

Most aren't painful, but you may experience mild discomfort. Sometimes a local anesthetic is used. Advances in flexible cystoscopy have made the procedures much easier to tolerate.

Do men with larger prostates have more-severe symptoms?

No. This is a common misconception. You can have a very large prostate with few or no symptoms, or a small gland with severe symptoms. That's because BPH is caused by growth in the interior of the prostate, not the outside part. Growth doesn't always affect the overall dimensions of the gland.

Does BPH increase my odds of having prostate cancer?

No evidence exists that BPH increases your risk of prostate cancer. The two conditions appear to develop independently of each other.

I've had several bladder infections in recent months. Could these be related to BPH?

There may be a relationship. BPH sometimes prevents you from completely emptying your bladder, and this can lead to infection. Talk with your doctor about testing that can determine the amount of urine left behind in your bladder after you urinate.

If I'm diagnosed with BPH, do I have to have surgery?

If your symptoms are mild and aren't too bothersome, you and your doctor may choose to engage in watchful waiting for the time being. If your symptoms become worse, you may consider either medication or a minimally invasive procedure to provide relief, in place of surgery. See Chapter 5 for details on treating BPH.

My father has BPH. Does that mean I'll get it, too?

Not necessarily. But because BPH does tend to run in families, your risk is greater than is someone's from a family in which BPH hasn't been diagnosed.

Chapter 5

Treating benign prostatic hyperplasia

Most men who seek treatment for benign prostatic hyperplasia (BPH) are bothered by persistent problems with the lower urinary tract. These include frequent urination, straining to urinate and inadvertent leakage of urine. Many of these problems occur because the enlarged prostate is blocking the urethra, causing changes in bladder function. (For more on signs and symptoms of BPH, see Chapter 4.)

Some men would rather put up with the inconvenience of BPH rather than treat it — hoping perhaps that their symptoms will improve or not worsen. But if your symptoms have reached a point where they're affecting your quality of life, causing anxiety and embarrassment, and preventing you from taking part in normal family life and social activities, it may be time to consult your doctor.

There are many treatment options for BPH. All treatments attempt to reduce the severity of your symptoms and restore the normal function of your urinary tract. Each option has certain advantages and disadvantages, and provides a different level of relief. The effectiveness of each option may vary according to your physical health, medical history and lifestyle needs.

This chapter introduces you to the treatment options for BPH and, in close partnership with your doctor, helps you assess the pros and cons of each form of therapy.

The severity of your symptoms and how bothered you are by them are key factors in deciding your best treatment option (see the prostate symptom index on pages 74-75). Depending on the size of your prostate and location of excess tissue, some treatment options may be more appropriate than others.

In addition, you must take into account the risk of side effects and the recovery time for each option. Your doctor can provide you with this information and recommend the best choices.

Watchful waiting

This option means you and your doctor have decided not to treat your BPH for now — your symptoms are likely tolerable. The doctor still examines you regularly and monitors your condition to see if the symptoms are improving, staying the same or getting worse.

Watchful waiting, also known as observation, expectant therapy or deferred therapy, is often the preferred approach for men with mild symptoms of BPH — for example, you're not bothered by getting up to urinate once or twice during the night. Watchful waiting may also be appropriate if you have moderate or severe symptoms — but only if you don't have complications, such as frequent bladder infections.

Most men who choose watchful waiting don't experience serious consequences for doing so. The advantages of this option are that you're not undergoing invasive treatment and not experiencing its side effects. Treatment generally doesn't cost anything more than the usual fees for a physical exam and perhaps some additional tests.

The risk of this approach is that your condition could quickly and drastically worsen or that other symptoms could develop, such as acute urinary retention. But this is uncommon.

With this approach, you may find that your symptoms improve for the short term, although in most cases the symptoms come and go. Some men will eventually decide to pursue more active treatment of their BPH.

While you're watching

Simple lifestyle changes can often help control the symptoms of BPH, and prevent the condition from getting worse.

Empty your bladder. Urinate all that you can when you go to the bathroom.

Limit beverages in the evening. Don't drink water and other beverages for an hour or two before bedtime to help you avoid nighttime trips to the bathroom.

Limit caffeine and alcohol. Caffeine and alcohol increase urine production and irritate your bladder.

Avoid bladder irritants. Certain foods may worsen symptoms in certain individuals. In addition to caffeine and alcohol, these include chocolate, highly spiced foods, acidic foods and artificial sweeteners such as aspartame.

Limit diuretics. If you take diuretics, talk to your doctor. A lower dose, a milder form or a change in dosage time may help. Don't stop taking diuretics without consulting your doctor.

Limit decongestants and antihistamines. These drugs tighten the sphincter muscle that controls urine flow through your urethra, making urination more difficult.

Stay active. Inactivity causes you to retain urine. Even light exercise can help relieve symptoms caused by BPH.

Keep warm. Colder temperatures can cause urine retention and increase the urgency to urinate.

Medications

Drug therapy is the most common approach that doctors may recommend to control moderate symptoms of BPH. Medications are also an option for men with mild BPH who are bothered excessively by the symptoms or who have decided against watchful waiting.

Two types of medications are currently used for BPH: Alpha blockers and enzyme inhibitors. Medications known as anticholinergics help relieve associated symptoms.

Drug therapy can significantly reduce major BPH symptoms. If these medications don't appear to be working over time, you may then consider surgery or a minimally invasive treatment.

Alpha blockers

This class of drugs was developed to treat high blood pressure, but they're also beneficial for other conditions, including BPH. They relax the sphincter muscles, which ring the urethra, helping to keep the passage open and making it easier for you to urinate.

The Food and Drug Administration (FDA) has approved four alpha blockers for the treatment of BPH:
- Terazosin (Hytrin)
- Doxazosin (Cardura)
- Tamsulosin (Flomax)
- Alfuzosin (Uroxatral)

Alpha blockers can work quickly and effectively to relieve BPH symptoms in many men. Within a week after taking the drug, you'll probably notice a much stronger urine flow and a reduced need to urinate, particularly during the night.

Alpha blockers are most effective for men with normal-sized to moderately enlarged prostate glands. They may not be appropriate if you're already experiencing serious BPH complications, such as significant urine retention in the bladder and frequent urinary tract infections.

Side effects are generally mild and controllable, including headache, dizziness, stomach or intestinal irritation, and stuffy nose. To reduce the risk, your doctor may start you on a low dose of medication and gradually increase the dosage. Some drugs are best taken before bedtime if they cause you to feel tired. You should take others on a full stomach.

Some men taking alpha blockers report feeling faint when standing too quickly (orthostatic hypotension). This side effect generally improves over time. Some of the newer, more selective alpha blockers may cause less dizziness than the older kinds do.

One occasionally bothersome side effect of alpha blockers is retrograde ejaculation, or dry climax. This occurs when semen flows backward into the bladder instead of forward through the urethra. Taking a lower dose or a dose every other day instead of daily may reduce the problem, but the trade-off may be less effective symptom relief.

Some alpha blockers are a good choice for individuals to control BPH and high blood pressure at the same time, which also saves some money on prescription drug orders.

Alpha blockers can lower blood pressure to unhealthy levels when taken with erectile dysfunction (ED) drugs such as sildenafil (Viagra), vardenafil (Levitra) and tadalafil (Cialis). ED drugs can interact in a similar fashion with other blood pressure medications, so don't take them together without checking first with your doctor.

Enzyme inhibitors

Enzyme inhibitors relieve BPH symptoms in a different manner than alpha blockers do. Instead of relaxing the sphincter muscles that surround your urethra, enzyme inhibitors help shrink the prostate gland itself. They do so by reducing the amount of dihydrotestosterone, a male hormone required for prostate gland growth.

Enzyme inhibitors include:
- Finasteride (Proscar)
- Dutasteride (Avodart)

If you have a large or moderately large prostate gland, enzyme inhibitors may produce significant improvements in your BPH symptoms. In men with moderate to severe symptoms, enzyme inhibitors may decrease the need for surgery and the occurrence of urinary retention. The drugs generally are not effective if you have a normal-sized or slightly enlarged prostate.

Enzyme inhibitors take a longer time to work than alpha blockers do. You may notice some improvement in urinary flow after several months, but it can take up to a year for complete results.

In most men, enzyme inhibitors produce only slight side effects. Some men may experience impotence, decreased libido and a reduced release of semen during ejaculation, but these side effects may subside when you stop taking the drugs, or shortly afterward.

Combination drug therapy

Taking an alpha blocker with an enzyme inhibitor can sometimes be more effective than taking one type of BPH medication alone. Not only can combination therapy effectively relieve symptoms and prevent them from getting worse, but also they can lower your long-term risk of acute urinary retention or the need for surgery.

The most tested combination is doxazosin and finasteride, but it's believed that any combination of alpha blocker and enzyme inhibitor is effective.

The side effects of combination therapy are assumed to be the same effects caused by each drug separately, but studies are needed to confirm this.

Once you start a course of medication, either alone or in combination, you'll likely continue using it over your lifetime for persistent relief. Some men may get quick relief from an alpha blocker while they wait for the enzyme inhibitor to take effect — often after several months. At that time, they may be able to stop the alpha blocker.

Anticholinergics

For years, urologists have prescribed a group of medications known as anticholinergics to reduce an overactive bladder and control urinary urgency. Anticholinergics relax the bladder's smooth muscle, increasing the amount of urine that your bladder can hold. The drugs also reduce pressure inside the bladder that creates the urgency.

In the past, doctors were reluctant to prescribe anticholinergics for men with BPH because an enlarged prostate obstructing the urethra could increase the risk of urinary retention if the drugs were administered. However, recent studies suggest that using anti-cholinergics in combination with other BPH medications can provide symptom relief without these concerns.

Anticholinergics commonly used with other BPH medications include:
- Darifenacin (Enablex)
- Oxybutynin (Ditropan)
- Solifenacin (Vesicare)
- Tolterodine (Detrol)
- Trospium (Sanctura)

Anticholinergics are available as tablets or capsules, but oxybutynin also comes as a topical patch (Oxytrol). Side effects may include dry mouth, dry eyes, constipation and drowsiness.

Heat therapies

Nonsurgical methods to relieve BPH use energy, such as microwave, radiofrequency and laser, to produce heat that destroys excess tissue in your prostate that's blocking urine flow.

These treatments don't destroy the entire prostate or even reduce its size by much. Instead, they work on shrinking the tissue around your blocked urethra, which will increase urine flow and decrease urine retention.

Heat therapies, or minimally invasive therapies, may be more effective than medication for moderate to severe symptoms of BPH, but also are more likely to cause side effects. Heat therapies may be less effective than surgery, but also less likely to injure healthy tissue or cause side effects.

Heat therapies are usually outpatient procedures. They generally cost less than surgery does and may also end up costing less than medications, if the drugs are taken over many years.

Microwave therapy

Transurethral microwave thermotherapy (TUMT) is the computer-controlled application of microwave heat to destroy the excess tissue in an enlarged prostate gland.

For the procedure, a flexible tube (catheter) is inserted through the penis and into the urethra. The catheter is equipped with a small microwave antenna that heats and destroys overgrown cells without damaging adjacent tissue. In some devices, water circulates around the antenna to protect the urethra from heat. A balloon at one end is equipped with a heat sensor to monitor the temperature.

TUMT usually takes about 45 minutes in an outpatient setting. Local anesthesia helps control pain, although you may feel some heat in the treatment area. You may also have a strong desire to urinate and experience bladder spasms. These responses are usually well tolerated and disappear as soon as the treatment is finished.

You may go home after you're able to urinate satisfactorily — usually the

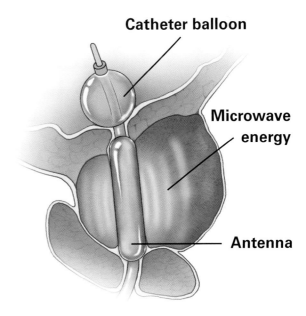

Catheter balloon

Microwave energy

Antenna

Microwave therapy

A catheter supplies computer-controlled heat to safely destroy enlarged prostate tissue. The catheter balloon at one end is equipped with a heat sensor to help control temperature.

same day of treatment. But several weeks may pass before you see a noticeable improvement in your symptoms — your body needs time to break down and absorb the destroyed prostate tissue. Painful urination may persist until the tissue is completely absorbed.

Many men require a urinary catheter for several days after the procedure. It's normal to have urgency, frequent urination and small amounts of blood in your urine during the recovery period. TUMT generally doesn't produce erectile dysfunction or incontinence.

TUMT works best for men with moderately enlarged prostate glands and moderate symptoms. It doesn't work as well if enlargement is primarily in what's called the median lobe, a posterior part of the prostate that can push against the wall of the bladder.

Because much of the prostate tissue remains, a need for additional treatment in the future is more likely than after standard surgery — either because the symptoms have returned or because they never adequately improved.

The procedure isn't recommended if you have a penile prosthesis or if you've had radiation treatments in the pelvic area or pelvic surgery. If you have a pacemaker or implanted defibrillator, consult with your cardiologist to see whether the device can be deactivated before the procedure.

Radiofrequency therapy

Transurethral needle ablation (TUNA), also known as Prostiva RF therapy, uses high-frequency radio waves to destroy excess tissue. This energy is delivered directly to the prostate by needles that are attached to a cystoscope threaded through the urethra. The cystoscope allows the surgeon to insert the needles at precise locations within the prostate before applying the heat treatment.

This outpatient procedure takes 30 to 45 minutes. Painful urination may occur, and many men require a catheter. It's not unusual to have blood in your urine for several days. You'll take antibiotics to prevent infection and mild pain medications such as nonsteroidal anti-inflammatory drugs (NSAIDs).

Other side effects may include temporary urine retention and urinary urgency. TUNA doesn't cause incontinence or erectile dysfunction. Most men can resume routine activities and sexual functioning within several weeks.

TUNA works best for men with mild to moderate obstruction of the urethra. The procedure doesn't work well for men with very large prostates.

TUNA is similar to TUMT in reducing urinary symptoms and improving urine flow. Typically, TUNA is less effective than traditional surgery but more effective than medications.

Laser therapy

Interstitial laser therapy (ILT) destroys excess prostate tissue with laser energy. A specially designed fiber-optic device is inserted through a cystoscope and into the urethra. The device punctures through the wall of the urethra into areas of the prostate containing the overgrown tissue. Once inside the prostate, the laser is activated to heat and destroy the tissue. Several punctures are usually needed to treat the entire area that's affected.

Similar to TUMT or TUNA, ILT works best for men with normal-sized or moderately enlarged prostates and who don't have poor bladder function. Because the procedure doesn't cause significant blood loss, ILT may be used for men who take blood thinners or who have a bleeding disorder.

Symptom relief generally must wait for tissue inflammation to subside following the procedure. Some men say their symptoms actually get slightly worse for a short while before they get better. Most men can resume regular activities within several weeks.

Surgery

Surgery was once the most common treatment for BPH. But with the development of other less invasive therapies, its use is on the decline. Today, surgery is usually recommended when nonsurgical treatments fail or if you have these BPH complications:

- Frequent urinary tract infections
- Recurring urine retention
- Bladder stones
- Blood in your urine
- Kidney damage caused by urine retention
- Inability to tolerate medical therapy

Surgery is still the most effective and lasting way to relieve the lower urinary tract symptoms caused by BPH. A procedure known as transurethral resection of the prostate (TURP) is the conventional standard by which all other treatments are judged.

So why is there less and less recourse to surgery in treating BPH? For one thing, surgery is more likely to cause complications and side effects than other treatments are, such as infection and bleeding. Also, surgery usually requires a longer recovery time.

But most men experience few long-term problems from surgery, although there's a risk of retrograde ejaculation, in which semen flows backward into the bladder. There's also a small risk of erectile dysfunction, incontinence and scar formation within the urethra.

Surgery is also not the best choice if you have a medical condition that would make undergoing anesthesia risky. This includes uncontrolled diabetes, cirrhosis of the liver, any major psychiatric disorder, and a serious lung, kidney or heart condition.

BPH surgery is performed by a urologist — a specialist in the reproductive and urinary systems. The four types of surgery for BPH include:
- Transurethral resection of the prostate (TURP)
- Transurethral incision of the prostate (TUIP)
- Laser surgery
- Open prostatectomy

Transurethral resection of the prostate

Transurethral resection of the prostate (TURP) is frequently used to treat moderate to severe BPH. In fact, it's one of the most common surgeries performed on men age 65 and older — although it's rapidly being replaced by the less invasive therapies.

During the procedure, you may be placed under general anesthesia or given a spinal block. The surgeon then threads a special instrument known as a resectoscope into your urethra. The resectoscope contains a light, valves for controlling irrigating fluid, and an electrical loop that cuts excess tissue and reseals opened blood vessels.

During the 60- to 90-minute operation, your surgeon uses the scope's loop to remove obstructing tissue one piece at a time from the inside of your prostate, creating an interior cavity. The tissue is carried by the irrigating fluid into your bladder, and then is removed at the end of the procedure.

You can expect to stay in the hospital for one to three days after surgery. You may have painful urination or a sense of urgency as urine passes over the

Resectoscope

Prostate gland enlarged by BPH

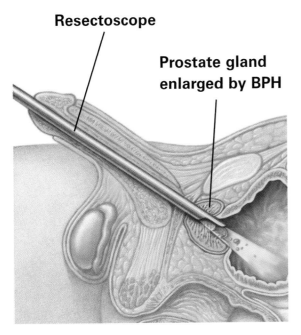

Transurethral resection of the prostate (TURP)

This is one of the most common surgical procedures for benign prostatic hyperplasia. Tiny cutting tools on the resectoscope scrape away excess prostate tissue and deposit the scrapings into the bladder.

surgical area. You can also expect some blood or small blood clots in your urine. You'll probably need to wear a catheter for several days. Most men are able to urinate on their own before leaving the hospital.

Symptom improvement should occur quickly. Most men experience stronger urine flow within a few days, and dis-

comfort should gradually improve over one to four weeks. You can do office work in about two weeks, and perform manual labor in four to six weeks.

TURP relieves BPH symptoms in nearly all men who undergo the procedure. It produces the greatest relief in men who have larger prostate glands and more bothersome symptoms. Even men with severe bladder damage often improve after TURP.

Occasionally, TURP can cause erectile dysfunction and loss of bladder control. These complications are generally temporary. Kegel exercises (see page 168) often help restore bladder control.

Other side effects of TURP are retrograde ejaculation and bladder neck contraction. A narrowing of the urethra, called a stricture, may occur that often can be remedied with simple stretching of the scar tissue, performed at the doctor's office. Occasionally, this problem needs to be treated surgically.

Additional treatment is uncommon, although some men may eventually require a second surgery — either because prostate tissue has grown back or not enough tissue was removed during the initial surgery.

Transurethral vaporization of the prostate. This procedure, referred to as TUVP, is a modification of TURP. It involves a special electrode that's inserted into the urethra by the resectoscope to vaporize excess tissue.

TUVP produces a nearly bloodless removal of prostate tissue. It also requires a shorter hospital stay and less catheterization time than does TURP. That makes this option useful for men at higher risk of complications, including those taking blood thinners.

However, TUVP is a more time-consuming procedure than is TURP. Each pass of the electrode makes underlying layers more solid and much harder to vaporize. TUVP is best limited to small prostates and shouldn't be used for very large glands.

Transurethral incision of the prostate

Transurethral incision of the prostate (TUIP) involves cutting or incising the prostate with a special instrument that's inserted through a resectoscope. Unlike TURP, no prostate tissue is removed. Instead, the surgeon cuts small grooves in the bladder neck — the location where the urethra meets

the bladder — as well as in the prostate itself. These cuts help relax the bladder neck and allow the urethra to expand slightly, which reduces the resistance to urine flow and makes it easier for you to urinate.

The procedure typically takes 20 to 30 minutes. You may be able to return home on the same day, or you may need an overnight stay in the hospital. A catheter is often necessary for one to two days after surgery. It may take three to four weeks for symptoms to improve. Generally, you can return to work in about two weeks, and resume sexual activity after several weeks.

TUIP may be a good option if you have a normal-sized or minimally enlarged prostate gland. It's also an option if, for health reasons, you aren't a candidate for more invasive surgery.

Outcomes for TUIP in men who are properly selected for the procedure are, in general, similar to the outcomes for TURP. There's also less risk of complications from TUIP than from TURP. Most men express satisfaction with TUIP, although some may experience only a small improvement in urinary flow. Additional treatment is more likely with TUIP than with TURP.

Laser surgery

Laser surgery uses a high-energy, low-penetration laser to destroy overgrown prostate tissue. Pulses of laser light are directed toward the interior of your enlarged prostate, which vaporize the obstruction and seal the area. The energy doesn't penetrate deeply, so surrounding tissue isn't harmed.

Several types of lasers may be used for this procedure. Each laser is slightly different in terms of intensity and delivery. One type of laser might be best suited for cutting, while another might be better for its coagulating effect on blood. If you decide to use the laser option, your surgeon and other specialists can recommend the best choice and answer your questions.

For the procedure, you'll be given general anesthesia or a spinal block. You may be allowed to go home afterward or you may need to stay overnight in the hospital. You may have painful urination and small amounts of blood in your urine for several days after treatment. Most men can resume routine activities and sexual activity within a few weeks. Laser surgery generally doesn't cause erectile dysfunction or prolonged incontinence.

Treatment often provides immediate symptom relief, moderately increasing your urinary flow and reducing the size of your prostate. Full symptom relief may take up to several weeks because of tissue inflammation. The inflammation can block urine flow and require the use of a catheter.

Treatment with laser surgery can be effective for many different sizes of prostates in men, ranging from small to moderate to very large. The procedure causes less bleeding than does TURP and recovery time is generally quicker. That makes laser surgery a good option for men who have platelet problems that slow blood coagulation or who are taking blood thinners.

Laser surgery to relieve BPH symptoms is relatively new, so its long-term effectiveness is unknown. Types of laser surgery include:

Photosensitive vaporization of the prostate (PVP). This procedure, also known as Greenlight PV, uses a potassium titanyl phosphate (KTP) laser to vaporize obstructing tissue. By doing so, the laser creates an interior cavity within the prostate that improves urine flow. PVP has fewer side effects and shorter recovery time than TURP.

PVP is generally an outpatient procedure that typically takes about 60 minutes to perform — depending on the size of your prostate. There is usually very little bleeding, although you may experience irritation when you urinate for several weeks after the procedure.

Most prostates may be treated with this technique, although occasionally the surgeon will elect to combine the PVP with a limited TURP procedure. For individuals with very large prostate glands, the PVP may be done in two separate operations.

A Mayo Clinic study indicates that participants have maintained symptom improvements after PVP over about a five-year period. Longer term data are still not available.

Holmium laser enucleation of the prostate (HoLEP). This procedure employs a holmium:YAG laser, which is well suited for cutting soft tissue and sealing blood vessels to reduce bleeding. HoLEP can be used on prostates of any size, even extremely large glands that might otherwise require open surgery.

With HoLEP, large pieces of prostate tissue are scooped out from their normal locations and pushed back into the bladder. Bleeding is controlled with the laser. The cut pieces are removed from the bladder with a special device called a morcellator, which grinds the tissue into smaller pieces that can be suctioned out through a cystoscope.

Similar to PVP, HoLEP is a safe, effective procedure that provides quick relief from BPH symptoms. A catheter typically is left in overnight and then removed the next day, when an attempt is made to urinate successfully.

Transurethral evaporation of the prostate (TUEP) and visual laser ablation of the prostate (VLAP). These are two of the original laser procedures developed for treating BPH. They've been replaced by more sophisticated technology and are seldom used today.

Open prostatectomy

Open prostatectomy involves surgical removal of the obstructing tissue in a prostate gland. The procedure is usually for men who have a greatly enlarged gland, bladder damage or other complicating factors, such as bladder stones or urethral narrowings. It accounts for very few operations for BPH in the United States, although it's performed more often in other countries.

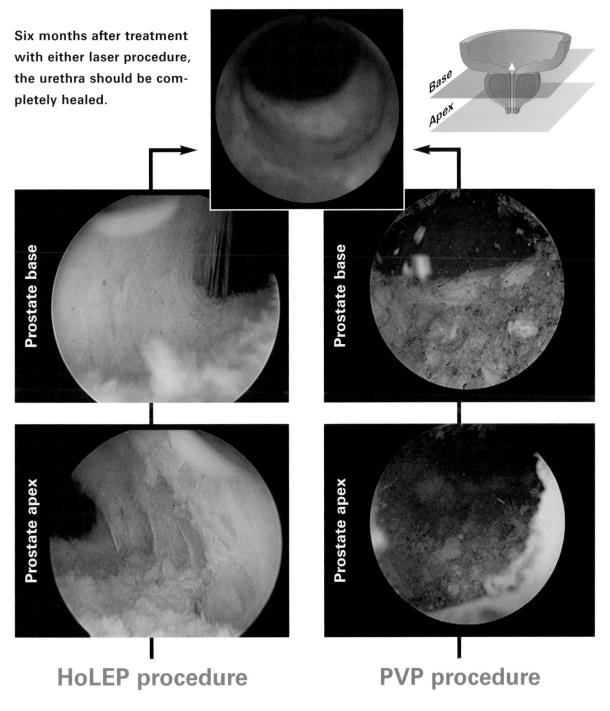

Six months after treatment with either laser procedure, the urethra should be completely healed.

Base

Apex

Prostate base

Prostate apex

Prostate base

Prostate apex

HoLEP procedure

PVP procedure

Two cystographic images show the HoLEP laser enlarging a narrowed urethra (the tip of the laser is the green semicircle). Loose pieces of tissue cut from the urethra are pushed into the bladder.

Two cystographic images show the cavity created in the urethra by the PVP laser vaporizing excess tissue that blocks the channel. Loose, tiny fragments of tissue are visible in the images.

The procedure is "open" because your surgeon makes an incision in your lower abdomen to reach the prostate rather than going up through your urethra. For the treatment of BPH, only the interior portion of the gland is removed. The outer portion is left intact, much as with TURP.

Open prostatectomy is distinct from radical prostatectomy, which is the surgical removal of the entire prostate gland due to cancer (see pages 128-132).

The open procedure is done under general anesthesia or spinal block, and requires a three- to five-day hospital stay. You'll need a catheter for at least three to seven days afterward. Most men can return to sedentary work in two to three weeks, and vigorous labor and sexual activity in about six weeks.

Open prostatectomy is often the most effective therapy for men with extreme prostate enlargement. Nearly all men who have this procedure experience significant symptom relief.

The side effects of this procedure are similar to those of TURP — erectile dysfunction, loss of bladder control and retrograde ejaculation — but their effects may be more pronounced.

Recovery from surgery

Depending on which type of prostate surgery you have, it may take several weeks to several months for a full recovery. During this time, avoid activities that involve lifting and jarring your pelvic area — such as operating heavy equipment or riding a bicycle.

Constipation can be a concern during recovery because of overly straining your lower abdominal muscles. To prevent constipation, eat plenty of high-fiber foods, such as fruits, vegetables and grains. Fiber softens your stool and makes it easier to pass.

Drinking eight glasses of water daily also helps cleanse your urinary tract and promotes healing.

Mechanical devices

Men with significant medical problems who are reluctant or unable to take medications or undergo surgery may have recourse to other options. These options include prostatic stents and urinary catheters.

Prostatic stents. With this procedure, coated metal coils are inserted into the urethra. The devices expand, like a spring, to widen the passage and hold it open. Tissue grows over the stents to hold them in place.

Stenting is done on an outpatient basis under local anesthesia and usually takes about 30 minutes. Symptom relief can occur immediately. The procedure produces little or no bleeding and doesn't require a catheter.

Most doctors don't consider stents a viable long-term treatment for most men. Some recipients find that the stents don't improve their symptoms at all, while others experience painful urination or have frequent urinary tract infections. These complications, along with the difficulties involved in removing the devices if they cause problems, have made stents a less popular treatment option.

Urinary catheters. A catheter may be necessary to manage urinary retention and incontinence. Some men have a permanent catheter installed with an external drainage bag that must be changed regularly. Other men learn to catheterize themselves when needed in order to intermittently drain the bladder. This helps prevent urinary tract infections and further damage to the bladder and kidneys.

Emerging treatments

No BPH treatment is perfect. They all have potentially damaging side effects. For this reason, researchers continue to seek out and develop new medications or new methods for treating the symptoms of an enlarged prostate.

Intraprostatic injections. Researchers are re-examining injection therapy as a way to deliver medications to the prostate — either via the perineum, rectum or urethra. This therapy has shown some initial benefits in treating lower urinary tract symptoms but long-term results are still unknown. It remains an experimental but promising minimally invasive option.

Alcohol ablation. Pure alcohol that is injected through your urethra directly into your prostate gland kills the targeted prostate cells without harming the surrounding tissue. Alcohol ablation isn't FDA approved and is considered experimental.

Botulinum toxin (Botox) injections. Recent studies show that injections of Botox into the prostate can relieve

A BPH shot?

Because benign prostatic hyperplasia (BPH) is such a common concern, new ways to deliver treatments also are being explored. Transurethral injection of various agents including alcohol, drugs, enzymes and botulinum toxin (Botox) may play a role in the future. Laboratory studies and preliminary trials in men suggest that the procedure is safe and effective. Mayo Clinic is among those institutions studying this form of injection treatment.

symptoms of BPH for six months or more. While results look promising, this procedure has not been approved by the FDA and researchers are continuing to study how botulinum affects the prostate.

New drug treatments for BPH. Experts are studying methods for improving the effectiveness and reducing the side effects of medications currently used to treat BPH, such as alpha blockers and enzyme inhibitors.

Researchers are also conducting studies on other, new means of removing, or ablating, prostate tissue, often by inserting different substances into the overgrown gland.

New classes of drugs are being developed that may be able to relieve lower urinary tract symptoms, either on their own or in combination with existing drugs. The new drug classes include:
- Muscarinic receptor antagonists
- Endothelin receptor antagonists
- Nitric oxide donors
- Purinoceptor modifiers
- Vanilloid receptor modifiers

These names don't refer to drugs; they refer to chemical pathways in your body. In theory, altering these pathways with medication may relieve the lower urinary tract symptoms — somewhat in the same way that pain relievers can alter the chemical pathways by which you feel pain.

Herbal therapies

Herbal treatments for BPH are available at pharmacies and grocery stores, and advertised over the Internet and in print. The most common herbal remedies used for BPH are:

- Saw palmetto
- Beta-sitosterol
- Pygeum

All three are commonly used in Europe to treat BPH. None has been approved by the FDA for use in the United States, but they're widely available here. The American Urological Association doesn't recommend using these remedies. Doctors have differing opinions about their use.

You may be seeking herbal treatments for a variety of reasons. You may be leery of the side effects caused by conventional medications used to treat BPH. Herbal remedies generally cost less than do standard medical treatments. They don't require a prescription or a visit to the doctor.

Be aware that herbal remedies haven't been adequately studied using scientific methods. Researchers aren't sure how safe they are or exactly how they work. Dosages, purities and ingredients available on the market vary considerably, and it's not known which dosage is most effective. Despite these drawbacks, growing evidence suggests that some of these therapies may merit consideration for symptom relief.

Make sure you learn as much as you can about the products and the benefits they claim to provide. Evaluate the benefits and risks or possible side effects. If you decide to use an alternative therapy, tell your doctor. Some herbal supplements may alter the effect of other therapies and medications. Others may create dangerous drug interactions.

Things to consider

BPH can be treated in many ways, and each option has its distinct advantages and disadvantages. No one can predict which treatment will work best for you and which one won't. The course of treatment you decide on is the one that you and your doctor have carefully considered and feel is right.

Keep in mind, the studies comparing the pros and cons of different treatments look at large populations of men. But you are one man — with your own concerns, health history, and levels of tolerance and discomfort. You must balance what you read with how you feel.

As you mull over the treatment options, it may help you to consider these key decision points and discuss them with your doctor.

How severe are your symptoms?

If the symptoms don't bother you and your condition isn't causing complications, you can probably wait to see if the symptoms will improve or worsen. On the other hand, if you have severe symptoms, organ damage or complicating factors, such as frequent urinary infections, bleeding or bladder stones, you may need surgery.

Treating anything in between depends on personal preference. Will you settle for small improvements, or are you hoping for more noticeable changes in your symptoms? Do you want immediate relief or can you wait? Are you willing to take medication daily? Will you tolerate some side effects?

How bothered are you by your symptoms?

This is a key question in the decision process that only you can respond to. You may have strong urinary tract symptoms caused by an enlarged prostate, but you may not be as bothered by them as another man with only moderate symptoms. If you're not bothered by your symptoms, there may be little or no benefit in treating them.

As a rule of thumb, for men with mild symptoms, watchful waiting is often the best approach. Men with moderate symptoms are often candidates for medication. Men with severe symptoms are typically candidates for minimally invasive treatments or surgery.

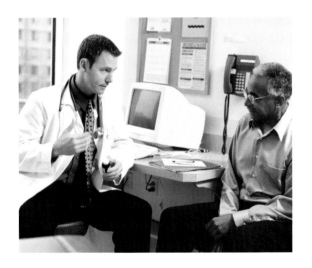

Are your symptoms getting worse?

Symptoms often come and go in men with mild to moderate BPH. But over the long term, they will tend to worsen. If you notice your symptoms getting worse, talk to your doctor.

One way to gauge if your symptoms are getting worse is to periodically complete the prostate symptom index (see pages 74-75) and evaluate any changes in your symptoms.

How big is your prostate gland?

Some treatments are best suited for large prostates, while others are more effective for smaller to moderately sized prostates. Therapies that are better suited for large prostates include:
- Enzyme inhibitors
- Transurethral resection of the prostate (TURP)
- Laser therapy (PVP, HoLEP)
- Open prostatectomy

Treatments that may be better for small to moderately sized prostates include:
- Alpha blockers
- Transurethral microwave therapy (TUMT)

- Transurethral incision of the prostate (TUIP)
- Transurethral needle ablation (TUNA)

What's your age?

The best treatment for a man in his 50s may not be the best for a man in his 80s. If you're younger, you may choose one of the minimally invasive treatments that provide long-term benefits, even if they don't provide immediate relief.

If you're older, immediate symptom relief from alpha blockers or surgery might be more important to you than long-term benefits. On the other hand, the older you are, the less suited you are to tolerate surgery. You may also be slower to recover from it.

How healthy are you?

If you have other serious health problems, you may not be a good candidate for surgery or recover from it as quickly. Surgery generally isn't recommended if you have:
- Uncontrolled diabetes
- Cirrhosis of the liver
- Serious lung, kidney or heart disease
- A major psychiatric disorder

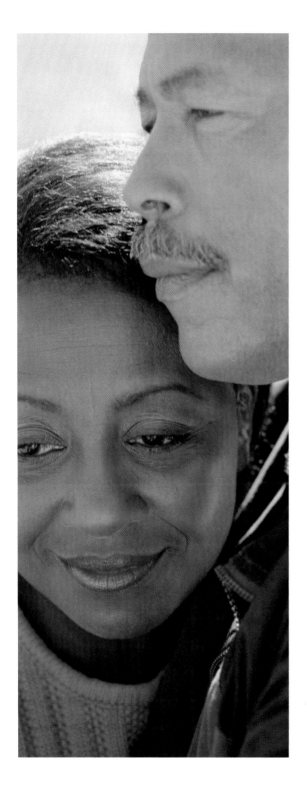

Some people aren't good candidates for medication because they don't tolerate a specific drug or class of medications.

Do you want to father more children?

If you want to father children, avoid therapies that may cause infertility. TURP, TUIP and open prostatectomy are most likely to cause retrograde ejaculation, in which semen backs up into your bladder instead of ejaculating from your penis. Less often, TUNA, laser surgery and alpha blockers cause this problem. Unlike erection problems, which may be temporary, retrograde ejaculation is often permanent.

Will you maintain your current sexual activity?

Surgery may damage nerves or blood vessels located next to the prostate gland, causing erection problems. Often, however, erection problems are temporary and normal sexual function, including the ability to have an erection and orgasm, returns after a few months.

Erection problems — even for a short time — are a concern for many men. Discuss this issue with your doctor before surgery.

Do the benefits outweigh the risks?

TURP — a surgical procedure — is still widely used to treat BPH despite the risk of more-serious side effects because it's excellent at relieving symptoms, it relieves them quickly and it rarely requires a second treatment.

Minimally invasive therapies are a trade-off alternative to surgery. They don't work quite as well as surgery does, and they're more likely to require re-treatment after several years. On the other hand, recovery time is generally quicker than from surgery, and less likely to cause serious side effects. They generally cost less, too.

As for medication, alpha blockers and enzyme inhibitors appear to offer long-term benefits, especially when used in combination. But they can cause side effects, you have to take them indefinitely, and the costs add up.

How long will it take to recover?

Recovery time varies with the treatment. If you choose medication, you don't have to worry about being laid up or missing work.

Minimally invasive therapies are often performed on an outpatient basis and ordinarily require only a few days' recovery time. However, depending on how quickly you're able to urinate on your own, you may need to stay in the hospital overnight.

Surgery for BPH requires a hospital stay. Plan for a two- to five-day stay if you have open prostatectomy. TURP and TUIP may mean a stay of one to three days. Occasionally, TUIP is done on an outpatient basis.

If you have an open prostatectomy, you may need to take up to a month off from work. For up to two months, you'll also need to avoid heavy lifting, jarring your lower pelvic area, or straining your lower abdominal muscles.

How experienced is your doctor?

Make sure that the treatment you and your doctor decide on is the best one for you — which is not necessarily the treatment your doctor has the most experience with. At the same time, in general, the more experience your doctor has with a particular therapy, the less risk of side effects and the greater your chances of a noticeable improvement.

Answers to your questions

Can treatment for BPH reduce my risk of getting cancer?

It may, depending on the treatment. A recent study showed that taking finasteride prevented or delayed the onset of prostate cancer by 25 percent in men age 55 and older. However, the same study showed that finasteride may contribute to an increased risk of sexual side effects.

Other BPH treatments don't reduce the risk of prostate cancer, with the exception of complete prostate removal. Even if you're being treated for BPH, you still need to continue regular prostate exams to screen for cancer. Some treatments for BPH, however, can identify cancer in its early stages. For example, unsuspected cancer is found during TURP in about 10 to 15 percent of men.

Is finasteride the same drug that's often used for hair growth?

Yes. Finasteride is used to treat both BPH (Proscar) and hair loss (Propecia).

The only difference is the dose. Proscar, for BPH, comes in a 5-milligram (mg) tablet. Propecia, for hair growth, comes in a 1-mg tablet.

If the first option I choose doesn't work, can I try another?

Absolutely. Conservative options, such as medication, are often the first choice of many men and their doctors. If conservative options don't produce satisfactory results, then you can move on to more invasive treatments.

Should I get a second opinion before deciding on a treatment?

Not necessarily. It depends on the confidence you have in your doctor and the therapeutic option that you choose. If you select a more conservative treatment, such as medication, or a minimally invasive therapy, your doctor has adequate experience with the therapy, and you feel comfortable with the decision, a second opinion may not be necessary. If you don't feel comfortable with your doctor's recommendation, it might be a good idea to consult another doctor.

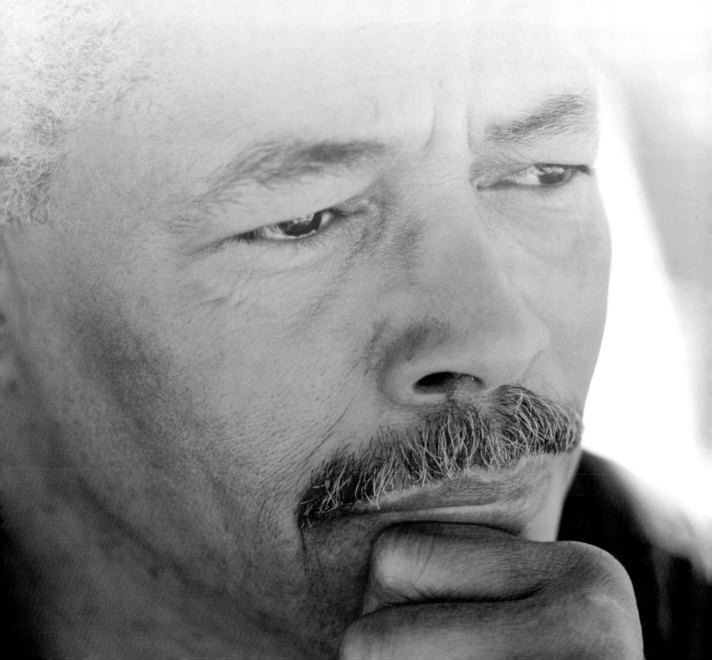

Part 3

Prostate cancer

Chapter 6

Learning you have cancer

Prostate cancer is the most commonly diagnosed life-threatening cancer in men in the United States. Each year, slightly over 186,000 new cases are diagnosed. Prostate cancer is also the second-leading cause of cancer deaths among American men — lung cancer is the leading cause.

As you age, your risk of prostate cancer increases. It's estimated that by age 50, about one-third of all men have some cancerous cells in their prostate glands. By age 80, this increases to about three-quarters of all men. The average age for men diagnosed with prostate cancer is 68.

Not all cancers act the same. Typically, prostate cancer grows slowly and remains confined to the gland, where it doesn't cause serious harm. Often, the cancer produces no signs or symptoms and is called latent. Some men may live long healthy lives without ever knowing of the problem, many times dying of something unrelated to prostate cancer.

Other times, the cancer does produce signs and symptoms, for example, an increase in the prostate-specific antigen (PSA) levels in your blood, or a firm touch during a digital rectal exam. These results generally warrant further evaluation and potential treatment.

What is cancer?

Cancer is a disease caused by abnormal cells that divide and grow uncontrollably. These cells can spread to normal tissue and destroy normal cell function. If not detected early, cancer often becomes life-threatening.

Cancer begins with damage (mutation) to the DNA in certain body cells. DNA contains a set of instructions that tells your cells how to grow, divide, develop specialized functions and eventually die. Normal cells frequently develop DNA mutations, but also have the ability to repair most of the damage. If the cells can't make the repairs, they typically die.

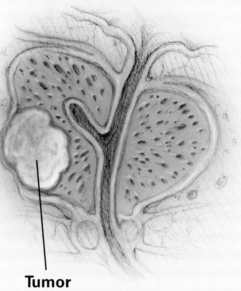

Tumor

The overall health of your body depends, in part, on this delicate balance between cell growth and development and the natural process of cell death (apoptosis). Sometimes, however, the process breaks down and certain mutations aren't repaired or eliminated. When that happens, the cells can grow without restraint and become cancerous. Mutations also cause these cells to live beyond their normal life span.

In some, but not all, cancers, the abnormal cells form small clusters (nodules) that develop into more densely packed, hard tumors. Cancerous cells can invade and destroy normal cells, either by growing directly into adjoining organs and tissues or by traveling to another part of your body through your bloodstream or lymphatic system.

Some forms of prostate cancer can be extremely aggressive, and these cancers quickly spread to other parts of the body. On average, an American male has about a 3 percent risk of dying of prostate cancer. This is because treatment of the disease can be effective when steps are taken early and because often, other illnesses ultimately cause death before the cancer.

The reasons why some prostate cells become cancerous and others don't, and why certain types of prostate cancer behave differently from others are unknown. Research suggests a combination of factors play a role, including family history, ethnicity, hormones, diet and environment (see "Are you at risk?" on pages 20-23).

However, this much is clear: Most men with prostate cancer that's detected while the cancer is still confined to the prostate gland can be cured. It's after the cancer has spread to nearby organs that treating the disease becomes more difficult — but not impossible.

Put simply, your goal is to catch prostate cancer early. That gives you more treatment options and a better chance of survival and preserving your quality of life.

Signs and symptoms

The problem with prostate cancer is that typically there's no early warning signs. The condition may easily go undetected until the cancer has spread beyond the prostate and has become much harder to treat.

When the signs and symptoms of advanced prostate cancer do develop, it's very easy to attribute them to another disorder. For example, many symptoms are similar to those you would experience with benign prostatic hyperplasia (BPH) — a much less life-threatening disorder.

Signs and symptoms of the lower urinary tract, which may be caused by a prostate tumor pressing on the bladder or urethra, include:
- Sudden need to urinate
- Difficulty starting to urinate
- Pain during urination
- Weak urine flow and dribbling
- Intermittent urine flow
- Sensation that your bladder isn't empty
- Frequent urination at night
- Blood in your urine

Other signs and symptoms that may signal cancer include:

- Dull pain in your lower pelvic area
- General pain in the lower back, abdomen, hips or upper thighs
- Painful ejaculation
- Painful bowel movements
- Loss of appetite and weight
- Incontinence
- Lethargy

Although these signs and symptoms don't always indicate prostate cancer, they should motivate you to contact your doctor for an evaluation.

Screening and diagnosis

Because prostate cancer frequently doesn't cause signs and symptoms, regular screening tests are critical for detecting the cancer in its early stages. Men who choose to have prostate screening usually begin at age 50. Consider earlier screening if you have a family history of prostate cancer or you are black. Most cases are now diagnosed in the first round of screening, before the disease has spread beyond the prostate.

Routine screening tests include a digital rectal examination (DRE) and the prostate-specific antigen (PSA) test. For a description of these procedures, see pages 26-28.

As described earlier, these screening tests by themselves are simple and not foolproof. However, because the DRE and PSA tests detect cancer in different ways, comparing the results may correct some oversight of the individual tests. That makes it more likely to catch the cancer in an early stage.

Biopsy

If the results of one or both screening tests are abnormal and your doctor suspects cancer, he or she may recommend that you undergo a prostate biopsy. With a biopsy, small tissue samples are removed from the gland and analyzed to determine if cancer cells are present. A biopsy is the only definitive way to diagnose prostate cancer.

To begin the biopsy, your doctor will insert an ultrasound probe into your rectum. The images help identify suspect areas and visually guide the procedure. The doctor uses a spring-powered instrument called a biopsy gun that propels a fine, hollow needle into the prostate gland to retrieve very thin sections of tissue.

Most often, the biopsy needle is inserted through the rectum wall into your prostate (transrectal biopsy).

Occasionally, the needle is inserted through the perineum, the area of skin between the rectum and the scrotum (transperineal biopsy). This is done when rectal access isn't possible or could cause bleeding or infection.

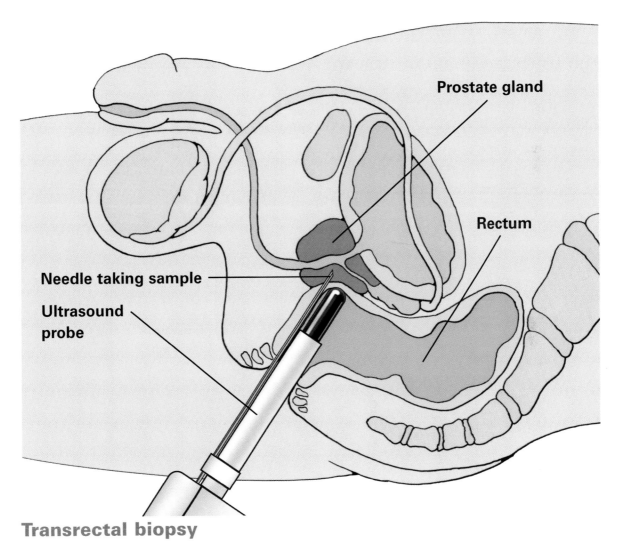

Transrectal biopsy

The biopsy gun, attached to an ultrasound probe, propels a thin needle into suspect areas of the prostate gland to retrieve small sections of tissue for analysis.

If an abnormal area is identified on the ultrasound image, your doctor will biopsy that area. If no suspicious area is noted, your doctor may take as many as 10 to 12 tiny samples from various parts of the prostate gland. Most samples will likely be taken from the outer portion of the gland (peripheral zone), where most cancer develops. (See the prostate zone diagram on page 16.) Sometimes, samples are also taken from the interior of the gland (transitional zone).

In preparation for the biopsy, you'll be given local anesthesia to reduce or eliminate any discomfort. Most men have virtually no pain during the procedure and usually don't require pain medication afterward.

You'll also be given an enema to reduce the risk of infection from digestive bacteria that might otherwise enter the needle incision. Antibiotics taken before and after the biopsy further reduce the risk of infection.

Common side effects of a biopsy include a small amount of rectal bleeding and blood in your urine for one to two days. Blood may appear in your semen, giving it a pink tint, for weeks to months afterward.

Biopsy samples are sent to a pathologist who specializes in diagnosing tissue abnormalities. The pathologist can tell whether cancer is present in the samples and how aggressive the cancer is.

Biopsy samples can identify specific cells that put you at high risk of developing cancer. Known as prostatic intraepithelial neoplasia (PIN), these abnormal cells are in the early stage of becoming cancerous. If PIN is found, additional biopsies may be recommended.

For men with more advanced precancerous cells, known as atypical small acinar proliferation (ASAP), there's a significant chance of finding prostate cancer on a later biopsy. If you have ASAP, your doctor may closely monitor your PSA levels and recommend biopsies at regular intervals.

Grading cancer

When a biopsy confirms the presence of cancer, the next step, called grading, determines if it's a slow- or fast-growing form. A pathologist studies your tissue samples under a microscope, comparing the cancer cells with healthy prostate cells. The more that

The Gleason grading scale

The Gleason grading scale runs from 1 to 5, with 1 being the least aggressive form of cancer cell and 5 the most aggressive form.

Grade 1. Cancer cells are small, similarly shaped and evenly spaced, like healthy cells.

Grade 2. Cancer cells are more varied in size and shape, and more loosely scattered.

Grade 3. Cancer cells are even more varied in size and shape, with some cells fused together into large, oddly shaped clumps.

Grade 4. Many cancer cells are fused into clumps that are scattered haphazardly and are invading nearby tissue.

Grade 5. Most cancer cells have gathered into large, scattered masses that have invaded nearby tissues and organs.

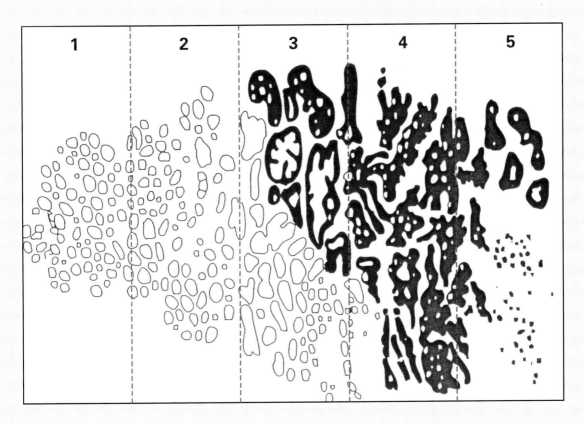

the cancer cells in your sample differ from healthy cells, the more aggressive your cancer is and the more likely it is to spread quickly.

The pathologist will assign numerical grades to the cancer cells, indicating how aggressive they are. But a single grade cannot reflect the complexity of this disease. The cancer cells will vary in size and shape throughout a single sample — some cells appearing more aggressive, and other cells appearing less aggressive.

The pathologist identifies the two most numerous and aggressive types of cancer cells in your sample — based in part on how the cells have fused or formed into scattered masses. Both types are assigned a grade, based on what's known as the Gleason grading scale (see page 113).

For example, the most common type of cancer cell could be given a 4, while the second most common type could be given a 3. The two numbers are added together to determine a total Gleason score — in this case, 7.

A Gleason score can help determine your best course of treatment. Scoring can range from 2 (nonaggressive can-cer) to 10 (very aggressive cancer). The lower the score the better. Scores between 2 and 4 likely mean the cancer is slow growing. There's about a 12 percent chance that it has spread to lymph nodes in the pelvis.

Scores between 5 and 7 indicate a moderately aggressive cancer — how aggressive will depend on a variety of factors, including how long you've had the cancer. There's about a 35 percent chance the cancer has spread.

Scores at the high end of the scale, from 8 to 10, mean the cancer is fast growing and has a greater chance of spreading. There's about a 61 percent chance the cancer has spread beyond the prostate gland to lymph nodes in the pelvic region.

Additional tests

Depending on your doctor and your cancer, one or more of the following tests may be performed to study whether your cancer has spread. Many men don't require additional tests and can proceed with treatment based on the characteristics of their tumors and the results of their PSA tests.

Ultrasound. This imaging procedure can be used to determine the size and shape of your prostate. Sometimes, it can indicate whether the cancer has spread to adjoining tissues outside the prostate. Typically, the test takes about 30 minutes or less. For more on the ultrasound procedure, see page 41.

Bone scan. This common procedure takes a picture of your skeleton to show whether cancer has spread to your bones. However, a bone scan isn't necessary in evaluating all cases, and generally it's not used when there's little reason to suspect the cancer has spread. For more on this imaging procedure, see page 49.

Interpreting a bone scan can be difficult in some people because the scan reveals more than cancer. However, doctors know that prostate cancer tends to spread first to bones near the prostate, such as the pelvis and lower spine — although the cancer can spread to any bone in your body.

In addition, doctors will look for isolated spots in one area of the body, which is more typical of cancer than are corresponding areas on both sides of the body — which may indicate, for example, arthritis in both hips.

Chest X-ray. An X-ray image can show if the cancer has spread to your lungs. For more on this procedure, see pages 42-43. Although prostate cancer usually doesn't spread this far, studies have shown that lung cancer has developed in many people with more advanced prostate cancer.

Computerized tomography. This procedure, commonly referred to as a CT scan, produces cross-sectional images of body tissue — each scan representing a thin slice of your body. A computer can gather the cross-sectional images together to form a detailed 3-D picture, allowing a doctor to view your prostate or other parts of your body from any angle. For more on this procedure, see pages 44-45.

A CT scan isn't necessary in every case of prostate cancer. As with a bone scan, your doctor may decide to order a CT scan only if there's reason to suspect that the cancer has spread from the prostate to surrounding areas.

Areas of new bone growth — from cancer, fracture, arthritis or infection — appear more dense than does old bone on a CT scan. In addition, this procedure can identify enlarged lymph nodes. When cancer begins to spread, one of the first places it goes to is your lymph nodes. The lymph nodes trap and try to destroy abnormal cells, causing the nodes to swell. Eventually, the nodes are overwhelmed by the cancer.

What a CT scan can't do is distinguish between cancer or another problem as the cause of abnormal lymph nodes. Furthermore, this procedure can't detect microscopic levels of cancer in normal-sized nodes. Therefore, CT scans are most useful when combined with other tests.

Magnetic resonance imaging. This procedure, commonly referred to as MRI, also produces a detailed, 3-D picture of your body. Instead of using X-rays and dyes to generate the pictures like CT does, MRI uses magnets and radio waves. For more on this procedure, see pages 46-47.

The primary value of MRI in the diagnosis of prostate cancer is to detect the spread of cancer to tissue outside the prostate gland, including lymph nodes and bone.

Lymph node biopsy. A biopsy is the best way to confirm that cancer has spread to nearby lymph nodes in the pelvic region. The biopsy is usually performed by a specially trained radiologist and can be done under local anesthesia by feeding a long needle into the lymph node through the skin. The sample is sent to a pathologist for laboratory analysis.

The procedure is most often used to verify test results indicating that the cancer is still confined to the prostate. If imaging tests show that the cancer has spread, then a biopsy usually isn't necessary.

There are three ways to remove cancerous lymph nodes:

- A radiologist uses a needle biopsy to remove a portion of the lymph node, guided by CT or ultrasound imaging. This procedure may be difficult when the lymph nodes are small and deep within the body.
- The surgeon makes a small incision in your abdomen and inserts a long surgical instrument equipped with a fiber-optic camera (laparoscope) to remove the lymph nodes.
- The surgeon uses conventional open surgery to locate and remove the lymph nodes through a larger incision. This method is most often performed when your doctor is also planning to remove the prostate gland at the same time.

ProstaScint scan. In this procedure, a radioactive molecule is injected into your bloodstream. The radioactive substance is attracted to any location in your body where cancer cells from the prostate have accumulated.

A radiologist specially trained in the procedure interprets images taken over several days. Wherever the radioactive material has accumulated in the body is where the cancer may be found. This test is highly specialized and often not required to evaluate and manage a case of prostate cancer.

Staging cancer

Grading indicates the level of aggressiveness of your prostate cancer. Staging determines if or how far the cancer has spread. Your doctor assigns a stage to the cancer based on careful study of all your test results.

This step is crucial because cancer confined to the prostate has a high cure rate. Once cancer extends beyond the prostate, the survival rate declines. The staging designation communicates to you and to health care personnel how advanced your cancer is.

Some men find staging information helpful for discussing possible treatment options with their doctors. Other men simply find the information overwhelming. If you have questions about your diagnosis or cancer stage, be sure to discuss this with your doctor.

TNM system

This is the most commonly used staging system for cancer in the United States. When the pathologist sends your doctor a report that stages your cancer, the report will include three capital letters — T, N and M.

- **T** stands for *tumor* and indicates the extent of the cancer in — and adjacent to — the prostate gland.
- **N** stands for *nodes* (lymph nodes) and indicates whether the cancer has, or has not, spread to nearby lymph nodes.
- **M** stands for *metastasis* (muh-TAS-tuh-sis), the medical term for cancer that has spread to other tissues or organs, such as bone or the lungs.

Each letter is followed by a number and perhaps another letter in small type. The numbers range from 0 to 4 and represent the extent of the tumor. The small letters go from *a* to *c* and indicate the location of the cancer.

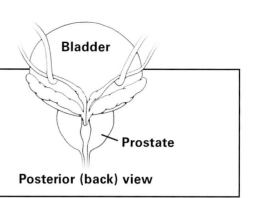
Bladder

Prostate

Posterior (back) view

Prostate cancer staging

Stage 1

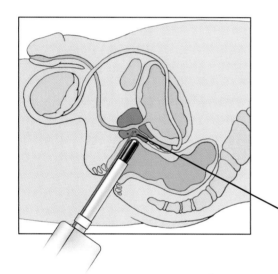

Cancer is detected following a test or procedure for another condition

T1a
Cancerous tissue is found in 5 percent or less of the removed tissue

T1b
Cancerous tissue is found in more than 5 percent of the removed tissue

T1c
Cancer is detected from a needle biopsy

Stage 2

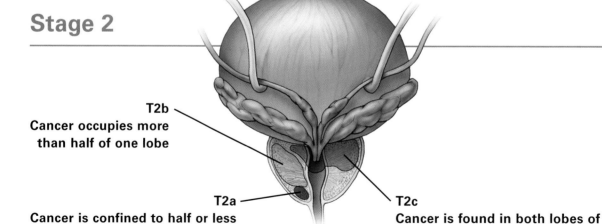

T2b
Cancer occupies more than half of one lobe

T2a
Cancer is confined to half or less of one lobe of the prostate

T2c
Cancer is found in both lobes of the prostate

Stage 3

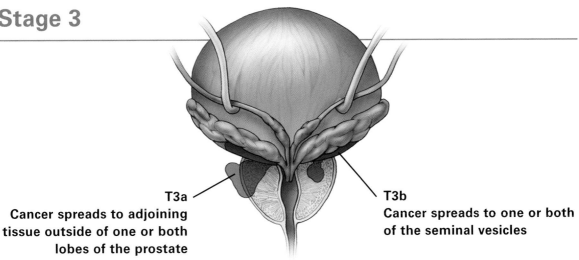

T3a
Cancer spreads to adjoining tissue outside of one or both lobes of the prostate

T3b
Cancer spreads to one or both of the seminal vesicles

Stage 4

This stage includes T4, any T1-4 and any N1-3, or any T1-4, any N1-3 and M1

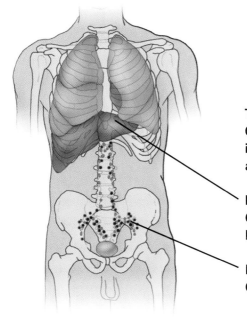

T4
Cancer spreads outside the prostate, which may include tissue in the bladder neck, external sphincter and rectum

M1
Cancer spreads outside prostate region to bones, liver, lungs and other organs

N1, N2, N3
Cancer spreads to nearby lymph nodes

Once the T, N and M results are known, the cancer is assigned one of four stages (see the illustration on pages 118-119).

Stage I. This signifies very early cancer that's confined to microscopic particles in the prostate that can't be felt during a DRE screening test.

Stage II. The cancer can be felt during a DRE screening test, but it remains confined to the prostate gland.

Stage III. The cancer has spread beyond the prostate to the seminal vesicles or adjoining tissue in the bladder.

Stage IV. This represents advanced cancer that has spread to lymph nodes, bones, lungs or other organs.

Some doctors use the older and more traditional ABCD system. In this system, A and B indicate cancer that's confined to the prostate gland, and C and D indicate cancer that has spread to other parts of the body.

Similar to the TNM system, each capital letter in the ABCD system is followed by a subcategory that represents details in the staging. Because the ABCD system has fewer categories, it's considered less precise.

What's next?

The decision tree on page 121 helps summarize the path you've had to follow for a diagnosis of prostate cancer. A suspicion that cancer has developed — often following an elevated PSA reading or abnormal DRE during regular check-ups — has led to a biopsy to withdraw small samples of prostate tissue.

If the lab finds cancer cells in your samples, the cells are studied for their level of aggressiveness and likelihood of spreading outside the prostate (grading). Further testing, including imaging tests, helps determine how far the cancer may have spread (staging).

This knowledge brings you to a critical juncture for deciding how to treat prostate cancer — has the cancer been caught while it remains confined to the prostate (localized), or has it spread beyond the prostate to other parts of your body (metastasized)?

Treatment for prostate cancer is different according to which path you take. Chapters 7 and 8 provide detailed descriptions of these treatment options and will help guide the decisions you may have to make with your doctor.

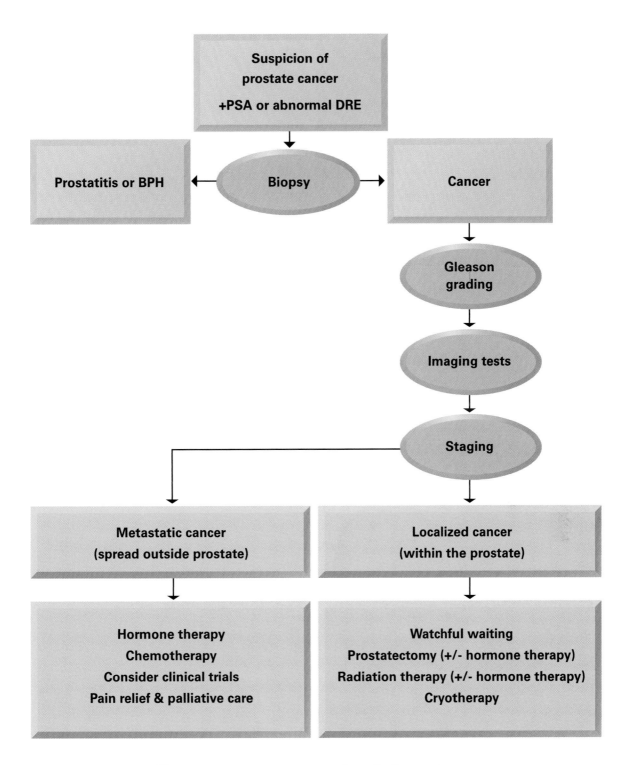

Prostate cancer decision tree

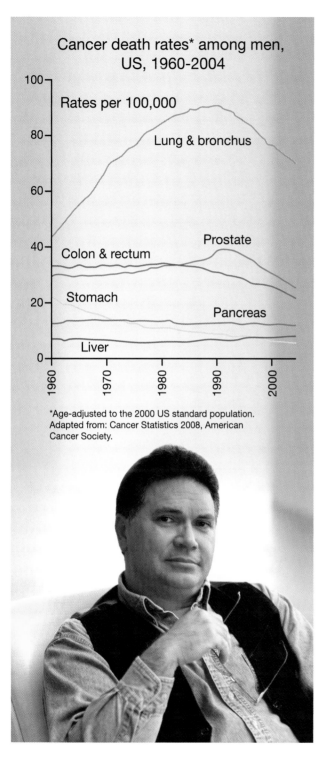

Cancer death rates* among men, US, 1960-2004

Rates per 100,000

- Lung & bronchus
- Prostate
- Colon & rectum
- Stomach
- Pancreas
- Liver

y-axis: 0, 20, 40, 60, 80, 100
x-axis: 1960, 1970, 1980, 1990, 2000

*Age-adjusted to the 2000 US standard population. Adapted from: Cancer Statistics 2008, American Cancer Society.

Surviving prostate cancer

The survival rate for prostate cancer has improved considerably over the past two decades. According to the American Cancer Society, the death rate for prostate cancer has dropped 34 percent between 1990 and 2004. Currently, there are approximately 25 deaths per 100,000 individuals (see chart).

In the mid-1980s the five-year survival rate for adult males with prostate cancer was 76 percent. That survival rate rose to 99 percent between the years 1996 and 2003, with professionals forecasting a continuing decline in mortality.

Today, about 91 percent of adult males with prostate cancer live at least 10 years, and 76 percent live 15 years or more. Black men continue to have lower survival rates than do white men.

It's hoped that survival figures will continue to improve if more men have regular digital rectal examinations and PSA tests to identify cancer during the early stages. For cancer that's diagnosed early and confined to the prostate, the survival rate is almost 100 percent.

Answers to your questions

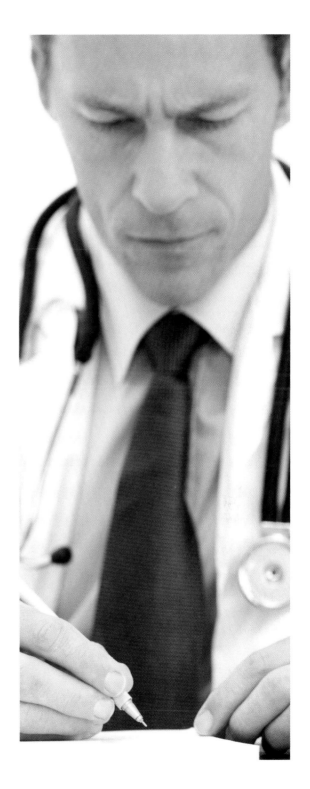

What are tumor markers?

These are substances made from cancerous cells found in your blood. When they exist in elevated levels, they may indicate the presence of cancer. During treatment and follow-up visits, your blood may be routinely checked for elevated tumor markers. PSA is a tumor marker for prostate cancer.

Is a biopsy the only way I can be sure I have prostate cancer?

Yes. Other tests, such as a digital rectal examination or PSA test, can suggest a strong possibility of prostate cancer. But a biopsy is the only way to be certain that cancer is present.

Can a biopsy be wrong?

When tissue samples are taken from a prostate gland, it's possible to miss the cancer. This is called a sampling error. A biopsy result that comes back normal isn't a guarantee that you don't have cancer. Sampling errors, however, are uncommon.

Can a biopsy loosen cancer cells, allowing them to spread?

No evidence suggests that this can happen. Cancer cells not removed in the biopsy stay within the tumor where they have been growing.

Why do I need to stop taking aspirin before a biopsy?

Aspirin and certain other pain medications thin your blood and can increase your risk of bleeding. Discontinuing these medications for a short period before and after a prostate biopsy will reduce your chances of serious bleeding from the procedure. The same is true for prescription blood thinners, taken to reduce clotting, such as warfarin (Coumadin).

Is it possible for a biopsy to cause permanent impotence?

No. Impotence that follows a biopsy is probably due to stress that often accompanies cancer diagnosis and treatment. In some cases it may result from temporary inflammation.

Can I pass cancer on to my wife during sexual intercourse?

No. Cancer cells won't escape from your body through intercourse. Even if they could, they wouldn't be able to grow inside another person because they're genetically coded for your body.

Chapter 7

Treatment options for prostate cancer

Learning that you have cancer typically produces fear, anxiety and sometimes panic. You may feel as if you need to make an immediate decision and begin treating your condition right away. However, because prostate cancer is often a slow-growing cancer, there may be no need to rush.

Give yourself time to sort through your emotions, set priorities and learn about the disease. Develop a strong relationship with your primary physician and the medical team that will be working with you. You'll need to trust their expertise and advice as you consider your treatment options.

You can gather information at a patient education library — if your local hospital or medical center has one — or at a local library. You can also visit well-respected sources on the Internet, such as the American Cancer Society, the American Urological Association and the National Comprehensive Cancer Network. While you're learning about prostate cancer, write down questions to ask your doctor before the two of you decide on a treatment plan.

At medical visits, you may find it helpful to take a family member or friend with you. There will likely be a lot of new information and unfamiliar medical terminology to sift through. Your companion can listen, take notes and help you recall the discussion afterward, including what issues still need to be resolved to take the next step.

Taking stock

There's more than one way to treat prostate cancer. And there's no one best treatment for everybody. The treatment of prostate cancer should be personalized to the circumstances, needs and values of each individual.

In fact, as you evaluate the pros and cons of various therapies, you may find that several treatment options may be available to you. Some men actually benefit most from a combination of two or more therapies. You'll need some time to consider the possibilities.

Which treatment you and your doctor choose will depend on several factors. These include how fast your cancer is growing and how much it has spread, as well as your age, overall health and life expectancy. In addition, you'll need to consider how much the benefits, risks and potential side effects of each treatment may affect you.

Watchful waiting

Because tests can now help detect prostate cancer at an early stage, more men have more treatment options earlier in the process. One of these options is to forgo immediate treatment and monitor your condition for signs and symptoms that the cancer is progressing.

This approach goes by several names, including watchful waiting, observation and expectant therapy. No medical treatment is provided — meaning medications, radiation and surgery aren't used. You keep a close watch on the cancer with regular blood tests and digital rectal examinations, performed about every six months. You may also need occasional biopsies.

If you're fairly young — in your 50s or 60s — and healthy at the time of diagnosis, your doctor may not recommend this approach. Because of your age, the cancer will have many years to develop, and even a small, slow-growing tumor may eventually need vigorous treatment. The cancer cells could spread so extensively that a cure becomes difficult or impossible.

However, if you're in your 70s or older and the cancer is small and slow growing at the time of diagnosis, watchful waiting may be an option. With regular, careful monitoring, you and your doctor can act quickly if the cancer does become aggressive and treatment becomes necessary to slow its growth.

A study by Swedish researchers suggests that, over the long term, there's little difference in the death rates among older men who followed watchful waiting and older men who pursued more aggressive treatment for prostate cancer such as surgery. Initially, the men who selected surgery were less likely to have cancer spread beyond the prostate and less likely to die of cancer than were men who chose watchful waiting. However, after six years, the survival rates for the two groups were similar.

Are you a candidate?

You may be a candidate for watchful waiting if:
- You're age 70 or older with a small cancer (Gleason score of less than 6)
- The cancer is slow growing and confined to one area of the prostate
- You're unable to withstand the side effects of treatment for reasons of age or health

- Your life expectancy is less than 10 years, because of another condition
- You're willing to assume the risk that you might miss the window of opportunity for a cure

Benefits

- You avoid side effects, such as erectile dysfunction or incontinence, associated with other treatments.
- You buy time to consider treatment options — it can take several years for a tiny tumor to double in size.
- It's the least expensive option, requiring only regular exams.

Risks

- The cancer can grow while you wait. Although rare, a slow-growing cancer may change into a fast-growing one. In such cases, the cancer may require more extensive treatment that results in more severe side effects than if it had been treated earlier.
- You may become what's called walking worried — always anxious about your condition and preoccupied with test results. Although more aggressive treatment has its risks, it may reduce the fear that you're gambling with your life.

Prostate surgery

Surgical removal of the entire prostate is a direct and effective means of treating a cancer that's confined to the gland. This type of surgery is called radical prostatectomy.

A majority of men in their 40s and 50s, and many in their 60s, choose radical prostatectomy. More men in their 70s prefer other options such as radiation therapy to surgery, and men in their 80s tend to choose no therapy at all.

New procedures and instruments developed during the past two decades have considerably changed how this type of surgery is performed. Surgeons use special techniques to completely remove the prostate and nearby lymph nodes while causing fewer complications and side effects.

The techniques try to spare muscles and nerves close to the prostate that control urination and sexual function. In the past, these might have been permanently damaged or severed. Better techniques also help control bleeding — resulting in less blood loss and the need for a transfusion — and improving safety and recovery time.

Radical prostatectomy is usually performed with general anesthesia, but you may request spinal (epidural) anesthesia — which numbs only the lower half of your body.

There are two primary open surgical approaches to the prostatectomy — retropubic and perineal.

Retropubic surgery

In retropubic surgery, the prostate gland is taken out through an incision in the lower abdomen that typically runs between the navel and the pubic bone, a couple of inches above the base of the penis. (See the illustration on page 17 as a guide to pelvic anatomy.)

It's the most common form of open prostate removal for two reasons. First, the surgeon can remove pelvic lymph nodes through the same incision. Second, the procedure gives the surgeon better access to the prostate, making it easier to spare the muscles and nerves that help control bladder function and penile erections.

The night before surgery you'll likely be given an enema or laxatives to clear your rectum of any fecal matter. This reduces the chance of infection if the rectal wall is punctured during surgery — an uncommon but possible risk.

Removing the prostate requires detaching the organ from the bottom of the bladder. In addition, the urethra is severed below the prostate gland, but above the external sphincter muscle that helps control urine flow. The vasa deferentia, which carry sperm from the testicles to the urethra, also must be cut. The seminal vesicles, which are potential sites for cancer spread, are removed along with the prostate gland.

Once the prostate is removed, the surgeon will reattach your urethra to your bladder. This reconnection allows you to urinate normally, although it may take several days to a few weeks — in some cases months — for your body to heal sufficiently for you to regain full bladder control.

After surgery, recovery in the hospital typically requires one to three days, and three to five weeks at home. A catheter is inserted into your bladder to drain urine. You'll need the catheter for about one to three weeks to give your urinary tract time to heal.

Lymph node removal. Through the incision intended for the prostatecto-my, the surgeon may remove the lymph nodes near your prostate and send tissue samples to a pathologist. Enlarged or suspect lymph nodes can be evaluated to determine if cancer is present. Results are often known within 15 to 30 minutes of removal.

Cancer in the lymph nodes means the disease is aggressive and more difficult to cure. If the lab results are positive and cancer is found, a critical decision will need to be made. Your surgeon may stop the procedure and close the incision without removing the prostate or may continue with the surgery.

A decision to proceed in light of positive lymph nodes depends on the number of lymph nodes involved, your age and health, and other planned treatments. The fewer nodes that contain cancer and the younger your age, the more likely your doctor will be to continue with surgery to remove the prostate and other cancerous tissue.

Risk of erectile dysfunction.
Depending on where the cancer is located, your surgeon will try to save the nerve bundles attached to each side of the prostate. These nerves control your ability to have an erection. Often, one or both of these bundles can be spared.

Men in their 40s and 50s who undergo this procedure are more likely to retain their ability to have an erection than are older men. For some older men — especially those not sexually active — the spared nerves still won't survive the shock of surgery.

If even one nerve bundle is spared following the procedure, it's still possible for you to have erections. If neither nerve bundle can be spared, normal erections are unlikely without treatment (for more on treatment, see Chapter 9). Even if your ability to have erections is lost, you can still have a normal sex drive (libido), your sensation is unchanged, and you can still have orgasms.

Regardless of the outcome, no fluid will be produced with an orgasm. That's because the structures that make and transport semen — the prostate, seminal vesicles and vasa deferentia — have been either removed or disconnected. The fact that you have dry orgasms has no effect on sensation, but it does mean that you won't be able to father children without medical help.

Perineal surgery

With this form of surgery, an incision is made between your anus and scrotum, which holds the testicles. There's generally less bleeding with perineal surgery, and recovery time may be shorter, especially if you're overweight. Unfortunately, the surgeon isn't able to reach nearby lymph nodes to test for cancer. This approach also makes it much more difficult — and sometimes impossible — for the surgeon to locate and save the nerve bundles attached to the prostate. That's why this surgery is less commonly used than the retropubic approach.

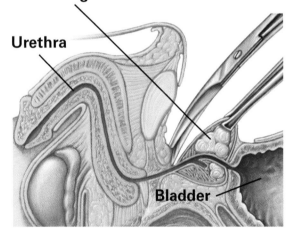

Prostate gland with cancer

Urethra

Bladder

Prostate removal

A radical prostatectomy involves removing the prostate gland (shown here with cancerous tissue) and seminal vesicles. The urethra, which is cut to allow removal of the prostate, is reattached just below the bladder.

After surgery

Before leaving the hospital, you'll receive instructions from your doctor about caring for yourself after surgery. The following may be part of your recovery routine.

A urinary catheter will be used to promote healing of the juncture where the urethra was reattached to your bladder. Follow instructions on catheter use carefully — they're designed to help prevent infection and blockage of urine. Drinking fluids is especially important in the weeks while the catheter is in place. This helps to keep urine flowing freely and reduce the chance of blockage.

List the medications you're taking daily on a sheet of paper. Include check-off spaces for doses and times (a.m., p.m. or both).

Try to avoid constipation by eating plenty of fruits and vegetables and avoiding red meat and pork for a couple of months. It's important not to have enemas or rectal examinations for a few months after surgery.

Don't become a couch potato during your recovery. Staying active is important, and walking is an excellent form of exercise. Movement helps prevent the development of blood clots in your legs — which can be life-threatening. See your doctor if you develop redness or tenderness in the area of a leg vein.

When your catheter is removed, you may experience leakage of urine. That's because it takes time for swelling to resolve in the pelvic muscles and for those muscles to regain their strength. You may need to wear diapers for several days, and an absorbent pad after that. Daily muscle strengthening exercises may be helpful. They can help reduce or eliminate your incontinence, but be patient — it may take a year or more. A good sense of humor also will serve you well.

Over time, incontinence can cause a rash near the tip of your penis. This is a yeast infection called balanitis. Your doctor can prescribe an antifungal cream. Wash your penis with soap and water daily and dry thoroughly before applying the cream, which clears up the infection and can help prevent a recurrence.

Are you a candidate?

You may be a candidate for radical prostatectomy if:
- Your cancer is confined to the prostate gland
- You're healthy enough to withstand the surgery
- Your expected life span is greater than the estimated life span that cancer would allow

Benefits

For cancer that's confined to the prostate gland, surgery is a very effective treatment. If cancer hasn't spread to organs and tissue in other parts of your body, it's possible to remove all the cancer cells and cure your disease.

Risks

- All major surgery carries some risk, including a low risk of death — which increases with age.
- You may have erectile dysfunction. This depends a lot on your age, the skill of your surgeon and the quality of your erections before surgery. If you had trouble achieving or maintaining an erection before surgery, the chances are greater that you'll have problems after surgery.

- You may have incontinence — at least temporarily. After the catheter is removed, nearly all men have some bladder-control problems for a few days. You could have problems for weeks, or even months. If so, medications and treatment can help improve bladder control.
- Recovery time can take from one to two months or even longer.
- There's a small risk of damage to your lower intestine or rectum. More surgery may be necessary to repair this damage.

Robotic surgery

Robot-assisted laparoscopic radical prostatectomy (RALRP) is a minimally invasive surgical approach to prostate cancer. Five tiny incisions are made in the abdomen through which the doctor inserts special instruments, including a long, slender tube with a camera on the end (laparoscope). The laparoscope provides the surgeon with a magnified view of the surgical area.

All instruments are attached to a mechanical device that is controlled by the surgeon — who guides the instruments while seated at a console

Robotic-assisted surgery

While performing robotic-assisted surgery, the surgeon sits at a computer console that's several feet away from the operating table (A). The robotic device has several mechanical arms equipped with specially designed instruments. Each mechanical arm features a flexible "wrist" that's capable of greater movement than is the human wrist (B). Typically, assistants are stationed at the operating table, making changes as needed to the instruments attached to the robot's arms.

The surgeon uses hand controls on the computer console to manipulate the robotic instruments (C). The tiny tools move in real time with the surgeon's hand movements.

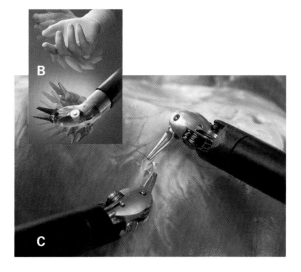

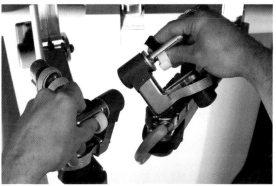

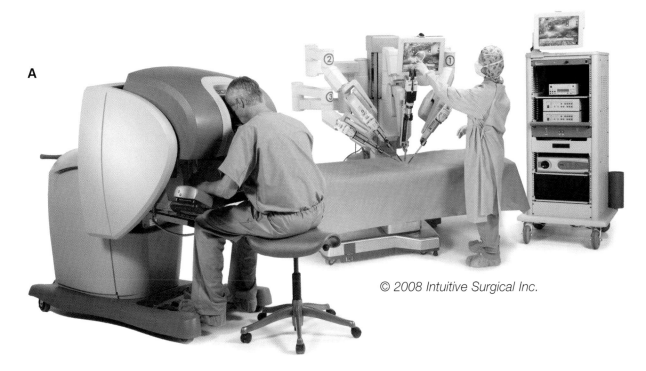

A

© 2008 Intuitive Surgical Inc.

equipped with a monitor for the laparoscopic images. Robotic techniques provide better precision and accuracy for removing the prostate and sparing the nerves around it.

This procedure is done while you're under general anesthesia. Surgeons experienced in the procedure can complete the operation in about two to three hours.

RALRP is the most common surgical procedure used to remove the prostate gland following a diagnosis of prostate cancer. Greater than 50 percent of prostatectomies are done with robotic assistance, and in some areas, that percentage is even higher.

However, RALRP isn't for everyone. Men with a lot of scarring from previous surgery, with a very large prostate and with distorted pelvic anatomy may not be suited for the procedure.

Benefits

RALRP generally provides greater precision and produces less bleeding, has a faster recovery time and usually requires shorter hospital stays (one to two days) than does conventional surgery. It can also result in less pain.

Risks

Because RALRP is a relatively new procedure, the time required to complete your surgery may be longer than with general surgery. Plus, the procedure requires general anesthesia.

The ability of the surgeon to feel the prostate and surrounding tissue may be important for decisions that need to be made during the procedure. For example, scar tissue, which may not show up on pre-surgical imaging, can greatly complicate prostate removal. While performing robotic surgery, the surgeon cannot feel the scar tissue.

Radiation therapy

Radiation is used to treat many different types of cancer and has been used to treat prostate cancer for decades. High-powered X-rays or other types of radiation are effective because they can interfere with cancer cells' ability to reproduce. Cancer cells are also generally more susceptible to the radiation's harmful effects than are normal cells and can be destroyed.

Radiation therapy is sometimes used if the cancer has not spread beyond the prostate gland or has spread only to nearby tissues. If the cancer has spread, radiation therapy may be used to help shrink the tumor — or to relieve symptoms when a cure is not possible.

External beam radiotherapy

When radiation is delivered from a device outside the body, it's called external beam radiotherapy (EBR). The radiation is most commonly generated by a machine — called a linear accelerator — that can focus a concentrated beam directly on the prostate gland.

Because the radiation can also damage healthy tissue next to the prostate, including the bladder and rectum, precisely locating the beam is necessary to reduce negative side effects.

Intensity-modulated radiation therapy (IMRT). This form of EBR uses high-powered X-rays to kill the cancer cells. For better accuracy, IMRT uses custom-made body supports prepared specifically for each person and for each treatment angle. These supports maintain the body in the same position from one visit to the next for treatment.

The supports help reduce the size of the area receiving a full dose of radiation, significantly limiting damage to adjacent, normal tissue and reducing side effects. Broader areas may be treated with X-rays if there's a concern that the cancer has spread beyond the prostate. Long-term outcomes for most men receiving IMRT are generally positive.

A first step in the procedure is to map the precise areas of your body that need to receive radiation. A radiation oncology specialist uses computerized tomography (CT) to determine the exact locations of the prostate and surrounding organs and to plan radiation doses. Computer software allows the specialist to rotate a 3-D image to find the best angles to fire the beam and deliver strong doses of radiation.

Treatments are generally given five days a week for about six to eight weeks on an outpatient basis. Each treatment takes about 15 minutes, although most of this is preparation time — radiation is received for only a few minutes. Anesthesia is not needed because there's no sensation of pain.

For the actual procedure, you'll lie motionless on a treatment table while the linear accelerator moves about you, targeting the cancer with radiation. To make sure the beams always hit the mark, the body supports hold you in the same position for each session.

Other, less high-tech measures may be taken to improve accuracy. You may be asked to arrive with a full bladder, which helps hold your prostate in the same position. Ink marks on your skin can serve as visual targeting guides.

Custom-designed shields in the machine are positioned to cover parts of your body such as the intestines, anus and urethra, protecting them from scattered rays. This precaution allows the technician to apply higher doses of radiation.

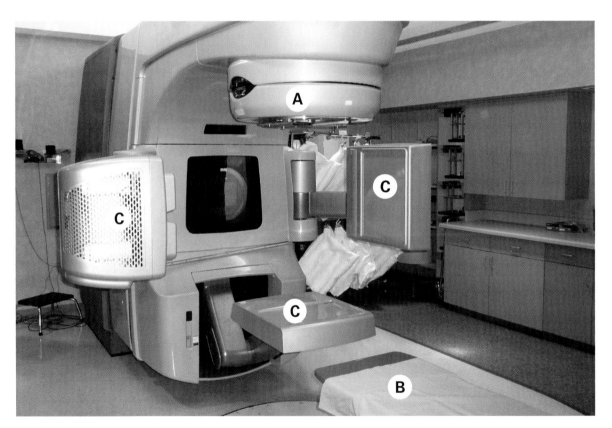

External beam radiotherapy

Radiation is delivered from a large, movable gantry (A) to an individual lying on the treatment table (B), which will be positioned below the gantry. Imaging devices (C) permit the radiologist to closely monitor the procedure.

A relatively new method uses small metallic markers to precisely locate the prostate before each treatment. These markers are inserted into the prostate using a method similar to that used to biopsy tissue before IMRT begins. Once implanted, imaging equipment uses the markers to determine the best position of the beam for maximum effect and least damage to surrounding tissue. Ultrasound imaging can also be used for more precise targeting.

Proton beam. This EBR method uses protons instead of X-rays to kill the cancer. Protons are parts of atoms that cause little damage to surrounding tissues but can effectively destroy cells when delivered in a focused beam. The protons travel through noncancerous

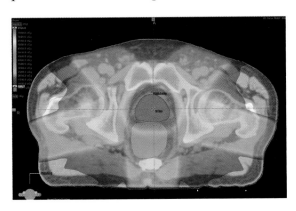

IMRT dosage

An axial CT image taken after IMRT shows the radiation pathways and dosage (green color) for the prostate (red color).

tissues and come to rest in the targeted area, where they deposit their radiation dose. This allows the therapist to deliver stronger doses of beam radiation.

Studies comparing the outcomes for treatment with protons with standard X-rays have not been completed. At this point, there's no evidence that protons kill more cancer cells than X-rays do. The advantage of a proton beam, if it exists, would be in reducing the damage to healthy tissue and limiting potential side effects.

External beam radiotherapy may be used at the same time that an individual receives hormone therapy (for more on hormone therapy, see pages 150-155). Studies have demonstrated that survival improves for certain men who have received both therapies, compared with men who received EBR alone.

Hormone therapy may be recommended for four months to two years — the duration depends on the cancer you have. Hormone therapy may precede the start of EBR but typically overlaps with it for a period of time.

EBR may be used after open surgery to treat the area where the prostate used to be — the prostate bed. This is done when an examination of prostate tissue indicates that small amounts of cancer cells may have remained after surgery. Such treatment will reduce the chance that the cancer grows back.

The radiation treatments are usually given no sooner than two to three months after open surgery and last from six to seven weeks. Radiation may also be given if your prostate-specific antigen level in your bloodstream starts to rise after surgery.

Radioactive seed implants

Another method of delivering radiation to cancer cells in the prostate is called brachytherapy (brak-e-THER-uh-pee). Rather than sending radiation from an external device, this procedure injects radioactive seeds, or pellets, directly into the prostate. The implanted seeds provide a higher dose of radiation than external beams do and cause less damage to surrounding tissue.

Brachytherapy may be used alone, but the procedure is generally done in combination with hormone therapy. Treatment with hormones helps shrink the size of the prostate, making the procedure easier to perform.

Hollow needles inject the radioactive pellets in and around your prostate. The needles pass through skin in your perineum, the area between your scrotum and anus. An ultrasound probe inserted into your rectum guides the placement. A template attached to the probe and held up against your perineum helps steady the loaded needles.

Depending on the grade of your cancer, the rice-sized seeds may contain one of several radioactive substances — called isotopes. The most commonly used low-energy isotopes are iodine-125 and palladium-103 (puh-LA-de-um). These seeds:

- Usually remain in place permanently, even after they stop emitting radiation
- Generally emit radiation that extends only a few millimeters beyond their location, and isn't likely to escape your prostate area
- Lose all radiation inside the pellet within a year

Between 80 and 120 seeds may be inserted — the total number depends on the size of your prostate. The procedure is done on an outpatient basis using either general anesthesia or a spinal block, which numbs your lower body. It typically lasts one to two hours.

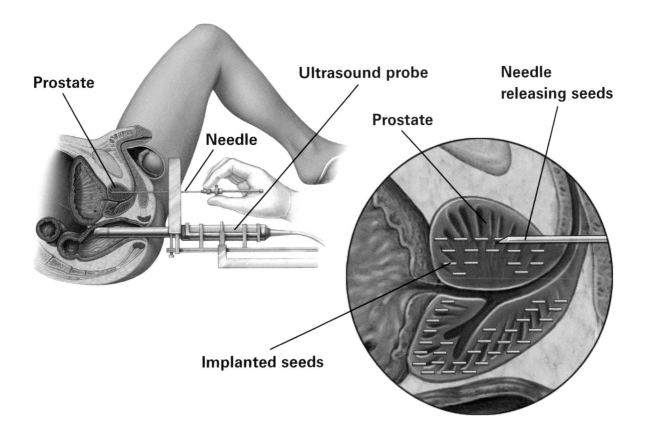

Prostate

Ultrasound probe

Needle releasing seeds

Needle

Prostate

Implanted seeds

Permanent seeding with iodine-125

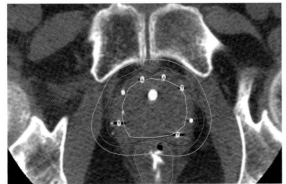

Temporary seeding with iridium-192

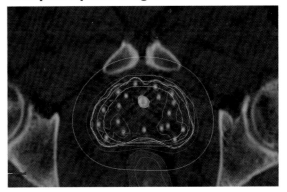

Permanent and temporary seed implantation

In the CT image on the left, each white dot (except the center one) indicates a seed of iodine-125 that has been permanently implanted in the prostate. The image on the right represents high-dose-rate therapy. Each white dot is a needle through which a source of iridium-192 will be placed temporarily in the prostate. Colored lines in both images represent a specially calculated radiation dose.

Another method uses a more potent substance called iridium-192 (ih-RID-e-um). Small amounts are left in the prostate temporarily, then are removed. This treatment is known as high-dose-rate (HDR) afterloading brachytherapy.

Permanent seeding requires one surgical procedure, while HDR requires two — after needles are inserted in the prostate, two to four treatments are given over eight to 24 hours before the needles are removed. The procedure is repeated two to four weeks later.

Studies have shown that brachytherapy has controlled cancer growth for five years in 90 percent of men who receive this treatment and for 10 years in 70 to 85 percent of these men.

The procedure is generally easier to perform on small or moderate-sized prostates, but men with larger prostates also may be considered for this treatment. Some men with very large prostates or a narrow pelvis will undergo hormone therapy to shrink the prostate.

As a precaution, doctors recommend that for the first few months after implantation with permanent seeds you avoid prolonged close contact —

less than two feet — with small children and pregnant women, who may be especially sensitive to radiation. Within a year, all radiation inside the pellets is generally exhausted.

Temporary implantation with iridium does not require special precautions because no radiation remains in you after treatment is completed.

Are you a candidate?

You may be a candidate for radiation therapy if:
- Your cancer can't be cured by surgery because it has spread outside the prostate
- You don't want surgery
- You expect to live longer than your cancer would allow you to live

Benefits

EBR and brachytherapy are both effective treatments for prostate cancer and can cure your disease.
- Both forms of radiation therapy are generally done on an outpatient basis. With brachytherapy, you may spend one night in the hospital.
- External beam radiotherapy is a noninvasive treatment that doesn't involve general anesthesia.

- Radiation therapy doesn't involve the rigors of open surgery. Recovery is generally less difficult and shorter in time.

Risks

- Radiation may affect sexual function by damaging nerves that control erections and arteries that carry blood to the penis. Most men don't have problems with erections at the beginning of therapy, but eventually many experience some complications. Your age and the amount of radiation you receive affect risk. Generally, the younger you are, the better your chance of retaining normal sexual function.
- Radiation therapy may produce urinary problems. The most common complaints are constantly feeling a need to urinate, burning sensation while urinating and urine leakage. Most problems are temporary and gradually improve a few months after treatment. You may need medication to treat these symptoms. The problems tend to be worse and last longer with brachytherapy than with EBR.
- Some men have bowel problems from EBR, including increased bowel movements, rectal bleeding, burning sensation around the anus and urgency to have a bowel movement. The signs and symptoms generally subside when the treatments are over, but for some men, may persist for a year or may require treatment. Rectal problems develop infrequently after seed implantation.

Cryotherapy

An alternative to surgery and radiation is cryotherapy (kri-o-THER-uh-pee), or cryoablation. The procedure freezes prostate tissue to kill the cancer cells. Doctors use a similar approach to kill warts, swabbing the abnormal growths with supercooled liquid nitrogen, which causes the cells to die. Prostate tissue dies in the same way and is absorbed by your body.

The procedure involves inserting several thin metal rods, each about 6 inches long, through the perineum and into the prostate. An ultrasound probe in the rectum helps your doctor position the metal rods.

Once the rods are in place, argon gas is circulated in the rods, which plunges the temperature of the rods to about minus 300 F. As tissue near the rods freezes, cancerous cells rupture and die. To protect the urethra, a catheter is placed inside the channel filled with a warming solution.

The entire procedure takes about two hours, with most of the time taken in positioning the rods. It takes about 30 minutes to freeze the prostate.

You can expect to stay in the hospital for one to two days — sometimes cryotherapy can be done on an outpatient basis. You'll probably be able to return to normal activities in about two weeks. It will take your body about nine months to a year to shed the dead cells. The procedure can be repeated if all the cancer cells aren't killed during the initial treatment.

You may be a good candidate for cryotherapy if:
- Your cancer is confined to the prostate
- You're not healthy enough to withstand surgery
- You don't want surgery or radiation therapy

Cryotherapy has been shown to control cancer confined to the prostate in 60 to 90 percent of men five years after treatment. Recovery time is short, and most men recover normal bladder function.

Cryotherapy doesn't always kill all of the cancer cells on the first try. It may have to be repeated. Other potential problems include:
- High risk of erectile dysfunction because the nerve bundles that control erections may also die.
- Trouble urinating for several weeks. Freezing swells the prostate, which squeezes the urethra.

Although short-term results look encouraging, long-term survival rates appear lower than do those with surgery or radiation therapy.

Emerging treatments

Initial study results suggest that the following therapies may prove to be viable treatment options for men facing early-stage prostate cancer. Further testing is required to better assess how outcomes for these treatments compare with standard treatments after five or more years have passed.

10 questions to ask your doctor

To better understand the best treatment options for you, ask these questions at the next visit to your doctor:

1. What options are available?
2. How fast will the cancer grow if left untreated?
3. Do you think the cancer can be cured with treatment? If so, what are the chances?
4. Which treatment would you recommend, and why?
5. How many times have you performed this procedure?
6. How soon before we know if the treatment has worked?
7. What are the risks of long-term side effects, such as erectile dysfunction or incontinence?
8. How soon is it possible to return to work?
9. Will any activities have to be restricted?
10. If a particular treatment doesn't work, are there other options?

New treatments for prostate cancer under development include:

- Prostate cancer vaccines, which are being tested to help your body's immune system recognize and attack certain proteins that are specific to prostate cancer cells.

- Targeted chemotherapy is under study that may be able to attack and destroy prostate cancer cells without killing off normal, healthy cells.

- Angiogenesis inhibitors, which are drugs that stop the growth of new blood vessels, may inhibit the growth of prostate cancer cells. Cancer cells need a steady blood supply to grow.

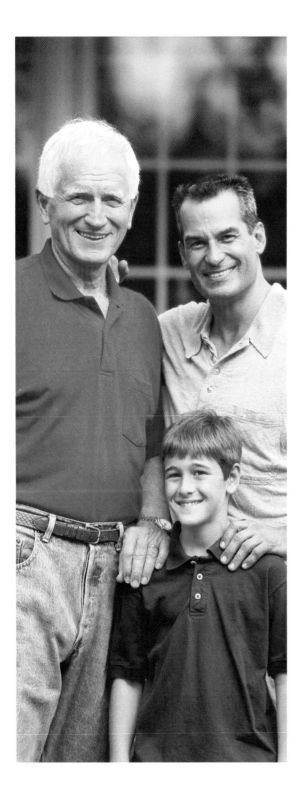

Things to consider

Choosing a treatment that will work best for you means weighing all the options in relation to your overall health, needs, values and lifestyle. As you make your decision, here are issues to consider and questions to ask yourself and your doctor.

How much time should you take to make your decision? Consider the aggressiveness of your prostate cancer — is it likely to grow rapidly? If so, it's important to make a reasonably quick decision and proceed with treatment. Slowly? Many prostate cancers are slow growing and may not require immediate treatment, so there may be no need to rush your decision.

What is the current state of your general health? Are there other conditions that may affect your health over the next few years? If you're young and relatively healthy, you may want to consider more aggressive treatment options, which may help you maintain that level of good health. However, if other conditions are affecting your health, you may choose less aggressive treatment because you're less likely to experience many of the long-term detrimental effects of prostate cancer.

How much of a factor is your age? Prostate cancer in your 80s is different from prostate cancer in your 40s. If you're in your later years, aggressive treatment may not extend your life and thus may not be warranted. You may elect to have treatment that is less invasive and has less severe complications.

A younger man may be willing to accept more aggressive treatment with more discomfort and significant side effects if that treatment offers a better chance of living longer.

It's important to consider your general outlook on life. Do you think of yourself as young and active? If so, you may find it worthwhile to consider the more aggressive treatments, regardless of your chronological age.

How much will your chosen treatment affect your lifestyle? Does the prospect of potential side effects — particularly impotence and urinary incontinence — bother you enough to sway your decision? Can your lifestyle accommodate, for example, a course of daily external beam radiotherapy?

Are you willing to commit to follow-up care? Your condition needs to be monitored after treatment — and the less invasive your treatment was, probably the more important that monitoring is. Are you willing to undergo routine blood tests, digital rectal exams and perhaps biopsies? Are you willing to schedule follow-up appointments with your doctor as necessary?

Once treatment ends, how much will you continue to worry about recurrent cancer? If you choose watchful waiting, how will you feel knowing that untreated cancer cells are inside your body? If you choose radiation — either seed implants or external beam radiotherapy — will you feel more confident that the cancer is under control or do you need the certainty of surgery?

How will your decision affect the relationship with your life partner? If you're married or in a relationship, you may want to think about how your decision will affect your partner. It's your life, but both of you will have to live with your decision.

Treatment for prostate cancer can be a life-changing event. An open, honest discussion before making a decision about treatment can help you both

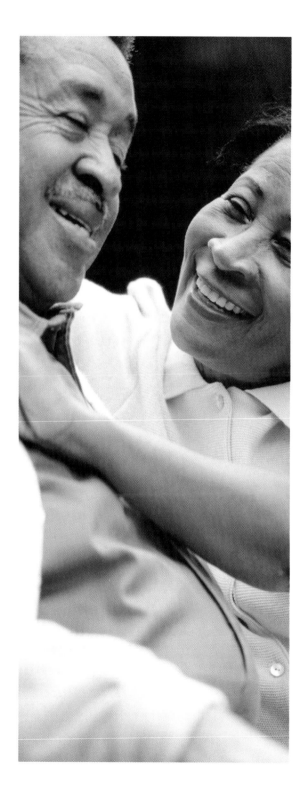

cope with the changes in your relationship if urinary or sexual dysfunction results afterward.

Discuss the trade-offs between the short-term and long-term effects. Your partner can help you talk through the value you place on benefits and risks.

Your decision has biological, psychological and social aspects, and may very well affect your sexual relationship and your daily life years after therapy is complete.

Is your doctor's experience and training having undue influence on your treatment decision? Make sure you and your doctor decide on the treatment that's right for you, not just the treatment that your doctor is trained in or has the most experience with.

How do you find a doctor who's skilled in this procedure? Before deciding on a particular procedure, talk with a doctor who can help explain the complexity of the choices you're facing and one who will listen to your concerns and values about health-related quality-of-life issues. You may feel more comfortable with making a decision after you've heard a second opinion.

Doctors who treat prostate cancer are urologists, radiation oncologists and medical oncologists. You may want to talk with a specialist in each of these areas because each may have a different opinion on how best to proceed.

If you choose a treatment option other than watchful waiting, select a doctor who has extensive experience with it. In many cases, your primary care doctor may be able to refer you to one or more specialists.

You can also get the names of specialists from a nearby hospital or medical school. Or contact the National Cancer Institute's Cancer Information Service at 800-422-6237. Any of these sources can give you information about cancer centers and programs supported by the National Cancer Institute.

Making your decision

You will likely face uncertainties in the decision-making process for treating prostate cancer. Both you and your doctor will deal with the fact that the tools for measuring the aggressive

nature of your cancer are not perfectly accurate. And it may be difficult to pinpoint the spread of cancerous cells to other parts of your body.

More uncertainty involves how well you're able to accept risk. You may feel comforted that the risk of urinary incontinence is only 5 percent for a particular treatment. But after the procedure, you'll be either zero or 100 percent continent, and that's an uncertainty that no one can predict. For more on incontinence and other side effects, see Chapter 9.

The best decisions come from taking time to gather all the information, thinking things over carefully, consulting with many experts and participating in the decision process. Your family and friends, as well as your primary physician, the medical team, and other cancer survivors, can offer support and encouragement. You don't have to make your decision alone.

Making a final choice may seem difficult, but you'll have done so based on a careful, honest appraisal of the facts, and with your best interests in mind. Whatever you decide, don't be discouraged. Prostate cancer is curable and even the most advanced cancer can be controlled, sometimes for many years.

Answers to your questions

Is surgery more difficult in some men?

Radical prostatectomy can be more challenging in men who are obese or who have an especially deep or narrow pelvis. A very large prostate also can be more challenging to remove. However, a skilled surgeon should be able to overcome these obstacles.

Isn't radiation harmful?

Radiation can be harmful to normal tissue if it's given in excess. That's why the amount you receive during radiation therapy is precisely calculated and controlled to minimize damage to healthy cells.

Can the radioactive seeds work their way out of the prostate gland?

Occasionally some seeds can get into the urethra and be excreted in your urine. This generally doesn't cause problems. Seeds may also infrequently become dislodged and travel through the bloodstream to other parts of the body, typically the chest and lungs.

The number of seeds that may migrate from the prostate is very small — less than 1 percent — and few side effects have been reported. A new type of seed that's built into an absorbable strand is designed to reduce the chance that seeds will migrate.

Should I get a second opinion before making a decision?

If you feel confident in your doctor and comfortable with your treatment plan, a second opinion may not be necessary. However, if you have concerns about your diagnosis, you don't feel confident in your doctor, or you don't feel comfortable with the proposed treatment, then you may want another opinion. If you're considering all treatment options, reviewing these options with different specialists is recommended.

Chapter 8

When cancer is advanced

How you and your doctor decide to treat your prostate cancer — and the challenges you'll face — depends on a very basic fact: Cancer that is detected early and remains within the prostate gland is often less aggressive and curable. Cancer that has spread to tissues outside the prostate has become a more advanced form and will be more aggressive and difficult to treat.

Prostate cancer in an advanced stage is also known as metastatic (met-uh-STAT-ik) prostate cancer. There may not be signs and symptoms, but the ones that appear most often include bone pain and weight loss.

Treatments that were effective with early-stage cancer, such as prostate surgery and radiation therapy, are no longer able to contain and destroy all the cancer cells. More organs and body systems are involved. The focus shifts to certain treatments that can help slow the growth of or even shrink cancerous tumors. Attention is also directed to symptom relief.

The fact that metastatic prostate cancer is more serious and life-threatening is not a reason to give up hope. There are many treatment options you can try that will allow you to live longer and enjoy a better quality of life.

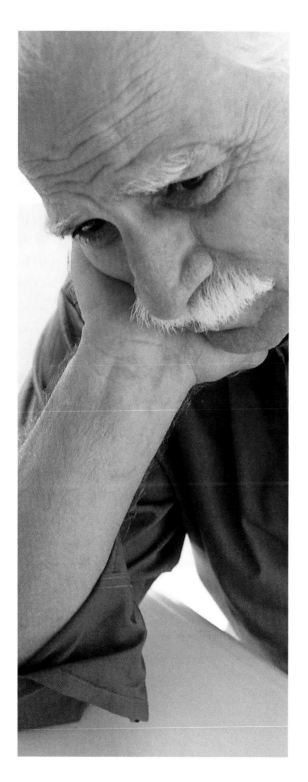

The options you have in fighting advanced prostate cancer include hormone therapy and chemotherapy. Several experimental therapies are currently in development.

Hormone therapy

Many prostate cancers are stimulated by the male sex hormones, or androgens — from the Greek words *andros* (man) and *gennan* (to produce). These androgens include testosterone, the main male sex hormone responsible for normal development of the penis and testicles, as well as other male features such as facial hair and musculature.

When you have prostate cancer, the circulation of androgens throughout your body and around the cancer cells in your prostate makes the cancer grow faster. A way of slowing the growth of the tumors would be to drastically reduce or cut off the supply of androgens to the cancer.

Hormone therapy — sometimes called androgen deprivation therapy (ADT) — uses medications or testicular removal to turn off the hormonal tap in one of two ways (and sometimes both):

- Stop your body's production of most, but not all, androgens
- Block androgens in circulation from getting into the cancer cells

ADT is so effective at shrinking tumors that it's being used in some early-stage prostate cancers, as well — in combination with surgery, cryotherapy and radiation therapy. Treatment helps shrink large tumors so that it's easier for freezing or radiation to destroy them or for surgery to remove them. And after more aggressive treatment, the drugs can help kill stray cells left behind at the tumor site.

Early use of ADT may also benefit individuals in which prostate cancer has been discovered in nearby lymph nodes at the time of a prostatectomy. The nodes may respond to hormone therapy without being removed.

On its own, hormone therapy isn't curative — that is, simply depriving prostate tumors of testosterone usually doesn't kill all of the cancer cells. It must be used in combination with another form of treatment to effectively rid the prostate of cancer.

There are two primary types of medication for ADT.

Drugs that reduce testosterone production

More than 90 percent of testosterone is produced by the testicles. Drugs can set up a chemical blockade, preventing the testicles from receiving messages from your brain to make the testosterone. These messages are carried by special brain chemicals.

Medications known as luteinizing hormone-releasing hormone (LH-RH) agonists can interrupt the message pathway. The medications are synthetic hormones similar to your brain's natural messengers. But instead of turning on the chemical switch to activate the pathway, they turn it off. Your testicles never get the message that they should produce testosterone.

Drugs typically used for LH-RH therapy include leuprolide (Lupron, Eligard), goserelin (Zoladex), histrelin (Vantas) and triptorelin (Trelstar).

These medications are injected into a muscle or under the skin. The action of the agonists endures for one month to a year, depending on the product used. You may receive injections for a few months, a few years or the rest of your life, depending on your situation.

Drugs that block testosterone use

Not all testosterone is produced in the testicles. Around 5 to 10 percent comes from the adrenal glands, located on top of each of your kidneys — and LH-RH agonists don't suppress this production. Medications known as anti-androgens keep this testosterone from acting on cancerous cells.

The drugs compete with testosterone for entrance into the cancer cells, eventually crowding out the testosterone. The most frequently used anti-androgens are bicalutamide (Casodex), flutamide and nilutamide (Nilandron). Depending on the drug you're prescribed, you take tablets or capsules one to three times a day.

Anti-androgen therapy can be used in combination with one of the LH-RH drugs, resulting in little or no testosterone getting to the cancer cells. Doctors refer to this combination as a total androgen blockade.

Intermittent use of drugs

Depriving prostate cancer of testosterone usually slows tumor growth but doesn't kill all of the cancer. Within one

to three years of ongoing ADT — which deprives the tumors of testosterone — the cancer often becomes resistant to the medications and begins to thrive without the male hormones. This is known as hormone-refractory prostate cancer (HRPC).

Once this resistance develops, your options to stop the cancer with hormone therapy are limited. Researchers believe that the continuous use of hormone medications may be the reason why the cancer adapts. Taking breaks from the medication might keep the cancer from adjusting to testosterone loss, or at least slow the process.

With intermittent therapy, you stop taking hormone drugs after prostate-specific antigen (PSA) in your blood drops to low levels and remains steady. You resume the drugs when your PSA rises again to a significant level.

In addition to reducing your risk of HRPC, other potential benefits of intermittent hormonal therapy include less cost for drugs and fewer side effects. A recent preliminary report showed that men receiving intermittent therapy were more likely to return to sexual activity than were men on continuous therapy. However, it's still too early to

know how the survival rate with intermittent therapy compares with the rate
with continuous therapy.

Are you a candidate?

If your cancer has spread beyond the
prostate gland, you may benefit from
androgen deprivation therapy.

Benefits

- Hormone therapy can slow the
  growth of prostate cancer and shrink
  tumors, reducing your symptoms
  and allowing you to live longer.
- Treatment may be stopped temporarily, allowing the return of normal hormone production.

Risks

- ADT lowers or eliminates the sex
  drive in most men.
- ADT can cause impotence, hot
  flashes and breast enlargement.
  Low doses of radiation can prevent
  the enlargement.
- ADT produces weight gain, often
  10 to 15 pounds, and reduces muscle and bone mass.
- Some of the drugs cause nausea,
  diarrhea and fatigue.

- ADT may increase the risk of diabetes and heart disease in men over
  age 65.
- In rare cases it causes liver damage.
- Most cancers become resistant to
  the medications in one to three
  years, on average.
- Some medications can cost hundreds of dollars a month and may
  not be covered by insurance.

With ADT, as currently practiced, about
50 percent of men whose prostate cancer has spread to other organs, such as
the bladder or rectum, live for five
years. About 40 percent of men live for
10 years. If the cancer has spread to
bone, this time is often shortened.

Recent reports have shown that men
who undergo hormone therapy for
prostate cancer may have a higher risk
of heart attack in the first year or two
after starting the treatment. Your doctor should carefully monitor your heart
condition and aggressively treat other
conditions that may predispose you to
a heart attack, such as high blood pressure, high cholesterol and smoking.

Testicular surgery

Surgically removing the testicles to prevent testosterone production was once

the standard treatment for advanced prostate cancer. It's still done, but hormone-blocking drugs have reduced the use of this procedure by providing what amounts to chemical castration.

Bilateral orchiectomy (or-ke-EK-tuh-me) is the medical term for testicle removal. Orchiectomy is as effective as androgen deprivation therapy in limiting testosterone production or use.

The surgery is often performed as an outpatient procedure using local anesthesia. The doctor will make a small incision at the center of your scrotum, the pouch that holds your two testicles. Each testicle is clipped from the spermatic cord and removed, with most of the chord left in place. Some men have an artificial implant placed into the scrotum during the surgery, to maintain a more natural appearance.

Are you a candidate?

You may benefit from orchiectomy if:
- You can't tolerate hormone drug therapy for health reasons unrelated to your prostate cancer.
- You aren't able to take daily medication as prescribed, or regularly visit the doctor's office for hormone injections.

Benefits

- The effects of orchiectomy are almost immediate. Within a few hours, the only testosterone left in your body is the small amount coming from your adrenal glands.
- Orchiectomy is performed on an outpatient basis.
- It's less expensive than the ongoing use of anti-androgen drugs.
- Side effects may be less intense than with hormone drugs, and the risk of complications is low.

Risks

- As with hormone drugs, orchiectomy reduces the sex drive in most men, and causes impotence, hot flashes and breast enlargement.
- You may feel less masculine and become depressed.
- It reduces muscle and bone mass, which can lead to osteoporosis.
- Though your cancer will probably go into remission for one to three years, it will almost certainly return, because cancer cells adapt to the absence of hormones.

After bilateral orchiectomy for prostate cancer, about 50 percent of men live three more years. About 25 percent live five years or more. Men with cancer confined to the pelvic area generally live longer — 50 percent to 60 percent live five years, and 40 percent live 10 years or more.

Chemotherapy

Chemotherapy is part of a first-line treatment for some cancers. In treating prostate cancer, chemotherapy is more often used in situations where other forms of treatment — including hormone therapy — have been unable or are no longer effective at stopping the cancer from growing and spreading.

As the name suggests, chemotherapy uses chemicals to destroy cancer cells. These drugs may be given with an IV, by mouth or by injection. First-line chemotherapy decreases PSA levels roughly in half for about 50 percent of individuals who take it, and causes tumor shrinkage in about 20 percent. Treatment generally extends the survival rate by several months.

Unfortunately, chemotherapy has unpleasant side effects because anticancer drugs are toxic to healthy cells as well as to cancer cells. Common side

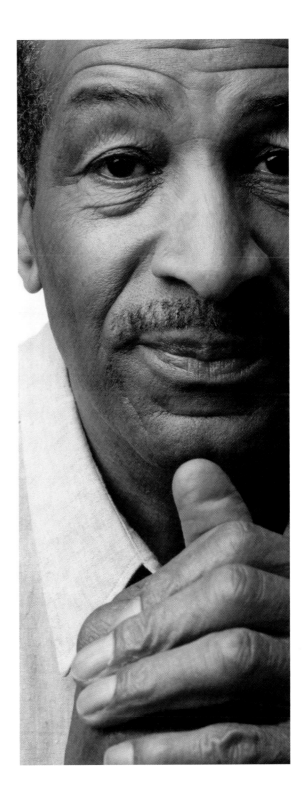

effects may include hair loss, nausea, vomiting, fatigue, changes in bowel function and lowered resistance to infection. The severity of side effects varies from person to person. In some, the side effects may be mild, while in others they're more pronounced.

Chemotherapy may sometimes relieve the symptoms of advanced prostate cancer, such as bone pain resulting from the cancer. It may also improve quality of life with regard to appetite, bowel function and physical comfort.

The most common chemotherapy agents are docetaxel (Taxotere) and mitoxantrone (Novantrone).

Are you a candidate?

Your doctor may recommend chemotherapy if hormone therapy is no longer working and your general medical condition is stable enough to try this treatment.

Benefits

Chemotherapy may relieve pain and other symptoms related to prostate cancer. The medications may slow tumor growth in some men and allow them to live longer.

Risks

Some side effects of chemotherapy may lead to discomfort. Other side effects may be more serious, such as a compromised immune system that can lower your ability to fight infection.

Experimental procedures

If traditional treatments are unable to control the cancer, your doctor may suggest that you consider participating in a clinical trial. Some trials involve traditional treatments, but in new variations or combinations. Other trials may be more experimental — some involving new medications.

To find out more about clinical trials, ask your doctor or visit the National Institutes of Health Web site at www.clinicaltrials.gov.

Gene and immunotherapy

Your immune system is capable of attacking cancer cells, but it often can't differentiate them from normal cells.

Researchers are attempting to genetically alter prostate cancer cells in the laboratory to make them more recognizable as foreign invaders. The altered cells would be injected into your body to help your immune system recognize and destroy all prostate cancer cells.

Cancer vaccines are another promising area of research. Intended to prevent cancer from developing or treat existing cancer, the vaccines are designed to strengthen your body's natural defenses against cancer, eliminate resistant cancer cells or prevent a recurrence once the cancer has been treated.

Another approach — still in theory — would be creating genes that are modified to attack only prostate cancer cells. The modified genes would be coded to switch on only when they came into contact with prostate cancer cells, limiting damage to healthy cells.

Experimental chemotherapy

Another area of research is focused on how prostate cancer cells can be made more sensitive — and vulnerable — to chemotherapy. This strategy has had some success in treating some forms of breast cancer.

Strategies for pain relief

Early-stage prostate cancer typically isn't painful. However, once the cancer has spread beyond the prostate to nearby bone — into the pelvic bones and progressively the spinal cord — it may produce intense pain. For reasons that are not clear, prostate cancer cells often migrate to bone tissue as they spread.

Pain isn't something you need to live with as you deal with prostate cancer. There are effective methods for getting symptom relief.

Treating local pain

Sometimes the pain from cancer is localized, or centered in a specific part of your body, such as your lower back. Your doctor may recommend various options for treating localized pain:

External beam radiotherapy. In this procedure, a high-energy radiation beam is focused on painful sites where prostate cancer has spread (for more on this therapy, see pages 135-138). It requires careful, precise planning that targets the cancer and reduces the damage to adjoining bone and tissue. Treatment is usually effective in completely or partially relieving symptoms.

Radioactive drugs. Doctors may also consider radioactive drugs, or radiopharmaceuticals, to help relieve symptoms. The radioactive elements samarium (Quadramet) and strontium (Metastron) are used in this targeted approach to localized pain.

Following an injection of either samarium or strontium, your bloodstream carries the radioactive element to your bones where it's absorbed. Cancerous bone tissue absorbs more of the radioactive substance than does healthy tissue — which helps concentrate most of the drug at the source of your pain. The radiation kills the cancer cells.

The benefits of radioactive drugs can last for several weeks or months, and sometimes even a year. If you find these injections helpful, you may receive more than one, but usually no more frequently than once every two months.

Depending on the dose given and the element used, your urine may be radioactive for the first few days after an injection and you must dispose of it in a hazardous waste container.

Following treatment, your white blood cell and blood platelet counts may decrease, putting you at increased risk of serious infection. Because of this, you'll likely undergo regular testing to monitor your blood counts.

Nerve stimulators. Although not widely used for pain associated with prostate cancer, transcutaneous electrical nerve stimulation (TENS) can offer relief for some men. Small electrodes attached to your skin near the pain site are wired to a small, portable battery-powered unit. Gentle electrical pulses travel to the electrodes and through your skin to divert your pain-sensing nerves.

Nerve blocks. An anesthesiologist injects numbing analgesic drugs into nerves at the pain site. This procedure works especially well if your pain is in a specific area where nerves can be identified and targeted.

Cryotherapy. This minimally invasive procedure can achieve good pain control by freezing cancer tumors in bone or surrounding tissue (for more on this therapy, see pages 141-142).

Surgery. Surgery may be required to correct or fix a fracture caused where bone has weakened due to cancer.

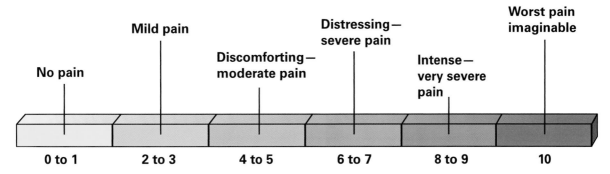

Pain scale

Use this scale as a guide when describing your perceived level of pain to your doctor.

The scale from left to right shows: No pain (0 to 1), Mild pain (2 to 3), Discomforting—moderate pain (4 to 5), Distressing—severe pain (6 to 7), Intense—very severe pain (8 to 9), Worst pain imaginable (10).

Treating general pain

Rather than being focused at a specific point, pain from prostate cancer can also be spread across a broader region of your body.

If you have general pain related to cancer, try to rate your experience of it on a scale of 1 to 10 — with 1 being no pain and 10 being the worst pain imaginable (see bar graph above). This will help you and your doctor assess the impact pain is having on your life.

Medications are often the first course of treatment for general pain.

Medications. If your pain is mild and no more bothersome than a headache, an over-the-counter (OTC) pain reliever may be all you need. If your pain is more intense, you may need a stronger prescription medication.

Opioids (narcotics) are commonly taken to relieve cancer pain. Some opioids are natural compounds derived from opium, while others are synthetic. Opioids include:

- Codeine
- Fentanyl (Duragesic)
- Hydrocodone plus acetaminophen (Vicodin, Lortab)
- Hydromorphone (Dilaudid)
- Meperidine (Demerol)
- Methadone (Dolophine)
- Morphine (MS Contin, Oramorph SR, others)
- Oxycodone (OxyContin)
- Oxymorphone (Numorphan)
- Propoxyphene (Darvon)

Opioids produce many side effects including mild dizziness, drowsiness, sedation and unclear thinking. Other side effects may include fatigue, constipation, nausea and vomiting. Ask your doctor about ways to manage these.

Opioids are powerful pain relievers. When taken in small amounts for short periods, they generally cause only minor side effects. But when opioids are taken in increasing doses for several weeks or months, these side effects can impair your ability to function in daily life. This may put your goals of pain relief and improved quality of life at cross-purposes. You and your doctor must work out the best approach when considering these drugs.

Another potent type of painkiller is tramadol (Ultram). Like an opioid, this prescription medication interferes with the transmission of pain signals.

Persistence pays off

The key to pain relief is working with your doctor to find an effective treatment. This may involve trial-and-error testing. If your first choice doesn't work, try another option. Keep trying until you find a therapy that controls your pain adequately and allows you to rest and be comfortable.

Many people think that pain is something they simply have to endure — that it can't be controlled. That's not true. Effective treatments are available. It's just a matter of finding the right one.

Other people worry that they may appear weak if they can't handle pain on their own. This also is a misconception. Advanced prostate cancer can produce severe pain because of the way it spreads to nearby bone, including the lower spine. Seeking relief from pain is not a sign of weakness.

Tramadol also triggers the release of natural hormones in your body that help decrease your perception of pain. Side effects are usually minor and similar to those of opioids.

Wide-field radiation. This procedure uses external beam radiotherapy (see pages 135-138) to treat a more extensive portion of your body, such as the entire pelvis and both thighs. Many men who receive this treatment say they feel better within two days. This number increases as lingering radiation from the treatment continues to attack the cancer cells. The downside, however, is that wide-field radiation can cause listlessness. It may also cause nausea if the abdomen is treated.

Radiofrequency ablation. Mayo Clinic doctors have found that a procedure called radiofrequency ablation can provide safe, effective relief for severe cancer-related bone pain when other treatments have failed. Radiofrequency ablation has previously been used to treat cancers of the liver and kidney.

In this procedure, a thin needle is inserted through the skin and guided to a cancerous tumor using computerized tomography or ultrasound. A high-frequency current is delivered through wires, or electrodes, to the tumor that creates intense heat, which deadens cancerous tissue. The therapy may also destroy nerves in the region that carry pain from the tumor site.

This treatment isn't permanent. The nerves often grow back, and the procedure may need to be repeated.

Complementary and alternative therapies

Some people look for pain relief from therapies that don't involve the use of medication or radiation — commonly referred to as complementary and alternative therapies.

These therapies range from massage to meditation to acupuncture to tai chi. The treatments aren't new — some have been practiced for thousands of years. But their use has become more popular as people seek greater control of their own health. Under careful supervision, one of these therapies may be of benefit in helping you manage pain.

Complementary and alternative practices are most commonly used in addition to conventional pain therapies. Some of these therapies are discussed in Chapter 12.

Answers to your questions

Can hormone therapy control prostate cancer for several years?

Yes. Many cancers adapt and learn to grow without the presence of hormones within about one to three years. But for some men, hormone therapy can control the spread of cancer for up to 10 years.

Will hormone therapy affect my voice or outward appearance?

No. Both your voice and outward appearance should remain the same.

Do I need to worry about becoming addicted to painkillers?

Many pain medications can be used effectively over many months and years without the danger of addiction. In cases of advanced cancer, the relief of pain, not addiction, is often your primary concern.

Chapter 9

Coping with complications

Prostate cancer is often a double blow. The first blow is learning to deal with the cancer. The second comes when you find out that treating cancer may leave you with incontinence and erectile dysfunction. The possibility of these side effects may be even more difficult for you to accept than your cancer.

Problems such as incontinence and erectile dysfunction erode feelings of self-worth. They can make you feel less in control and independent. It's too easy to convince yourself that the causes are "all in your head" — problems that can be resolved if only you draw on extra reserves of inner strength.

Acknowledging a condition such as incontinence or erectile dysfunction, even in private discussions with your doctor and health care team, may feel awkward. In fact, these side effects are not uncommon and affect many men dealing with prostate cancer.

Fortunately, when these side effects are part of prostate cancer treatment, they're often temporary — and even when they are permanent, they don't need to be devastating. Your doctor can offer good advice and support. Various treatments can help you effectively manage the complications and maintain a good quality of life.

Controlling incontinence

Urinary incontinence is the inability to control the flow of urine from your bladder, resulting in accidental and untimely leakage.

Incontinence is often a symptom of an underlying condition, which usually can and should be treated. It can also be a result of procedures or medications used to treat a condition, such as what may happen after certain types of surgery or radiation therapy for prostate cancer. The incontinence may subside when treatment ends.

Long-term incontinence after prostate cancer treatment is not common. But when it does persist, it can be extremely frustrating and embarrassing. You may stop exercising, stop going out socially or even resist the urge to laugh because you're afraid of accidentally wetting yourself.

Like many men, you may be too embarrassed to ask for help. Perhaps, you think incontinence is simply the price you pay for having prostate cancer — and that you'll just learn to live with it. That's not true. Incontinence can often be successfully treated.

For the urinary system to function properly, a complex network of muscles and nerves must work together harmoniously. Except when you're urinating, your bladder muscle stays relaxed so that it can expand to store urine. The relaxed bladder is supported by muscles located in your lower pelvis (pelvic floor muscles). Your bladder and pelvic floor muscles communicate with each other to help hold urine in the bladder without leaking.

Also helping to control urine flow is a ring of muscle around the opening at the base of the bladder, called the internal urinary sphincter. The sphincter's ability to contract around the urethra to close it, or relax to open it, also depends on involuntary pelvic floor muscles.

Treatments for prostate cancer — surgery, radiation and cryotherapy — can affect the pelvic floor muscles and the nerves that control them, producing incontinence. Often, though not always, the incontinence is temporary and healing occurs over weeks or months as the muscles slowly regain their strength and their ability to control urine flow.

What's a urethral stricture?

A urethral stricture is a narrowing of the urethra, which may occur in people who have had a radical prostatectomy. When your prostate is removed, the upper portion of the urethra is reattached to the bottom of your bladder. This restores the urinary channel, which previously had been surrounded by the prostate. Sometimes, scar tissue forms in the area where the urethra and bladder were reattached, causing the urethra to narrow.

Usually, the first line of treatment is to stretch the urethra by dilating it with a thin instrument that's inserted into the urethra. This is the simplest and safest approach. Occasionally, the stricture needs to be opened surgically. In some people, these procedures must be repeated more than once because of re-narrowing. If the stricture is severe, your doctor may suggest laser treatment to vaporize the scar tissue.

Types of incontinence

Urinary incontinence may be divided into four major categories:

Stress. This type is caused by physical stress on the bladder. Urine leaks occur with bursts of activity that put intense pressure on the bladder, such as lifting a heavy object, swinging a golf club, sneezing or laughing hard.

Urge. With this type, you feel an immediate, intense urge to urinate and you may wet yourself before getting to the bathroom. Your body may give you a warning of only seconds. This happens due to an overactive bladder, which contracts too often and at inappropriate times — namely when your bladder isn't full — trying to expel the urine. Your brain gets the message that you have to go — now.

Overflow. With this type, you're unable to empty your bladder completely, leading to urine backup. The backup builds pressure that exceeds your bladder's capacity to hold fluid. You frequently dribble small amounts of urine throughout the day. You may feel as if you never completely empty your bladder — or that you need to empty your bladder but can't. When you try to urinate, you may have trouble getting started and may produce only a weak stream of urine. This type is common in men with bladder damage, blocked urethra, urethral stricture or prostate problems.

Urodynamic testing

If you have a problem with urinary incontinence, your doctor may perform a series of diagnostic tests to determine the type of incontinence you have and how best to treat it. These tests include:

Cystography. A detailed X-ray examination of your urethra and bladder that uses contrast dye to enhance the images.

Cystometrography. A procedure that measures varying pressure levels as your bladder fills with, and then releases, urine.

Cystoscopy. A study of the inner surface of the urinary tract and the function of your urinary sphincter muscle by inserting a thin, flexible tube equipped with a light and lens into your urethra.

Uroflowometry. This test measures the force of urine flow, including how much urine you release, how fast urine leaves the penis, and how long it takes to empty your bladder.

Mixed. This is a combination of two or more types of incontinence, typically stress incontinence and urge incontinence. You have signs and symptoms of both, but usually one type will be more bothersome than the other is. The cause of the two forms may or may not be related. Men who've had their prostate glands removed or who've had surgery for enlarged prostates can develop mixed incontinence.

Treatment

For most men, urinary incontinence after prostate surgery is temporary as normal bladder control gradually returns. You'll need to use a catheter for one to three weeks immediately after the procedure while the swollen tissues heal. Incontinence may occur when the catheter is removed and while the pelvic floor muscles are still weak.

You may need to wear absorbent pads or underwear for a short time, as you regain control of urine flow. Most men see a noticeable reduction in urine leakage within a short time, as the muscles and nerves strengthen.

For some men, incontinence becomes chronic. If other treatment options are necessary, behavioral techniques, med-

ications, devices and surgery may be considered. Often, your doctor will suggest the least invasive treatment first, and move to other options if this is not successful.

Behavior techniques. Modifications to your behavior include timed urination, that is, going to the bathroom according to the clock rather than waiting for the urge to go. You go to the toilet on a planned basis — usually every hour or so at the start, and then try to build to longer intervals to retrain the bladder.

You may adjust your dietary habits, for example, learning to avoid alcohol, caffeine and certain acidic foods that irritate your bladder. For some individuals, reducing liquid consumption before bedtime is all that's needed. Losing weight also may eliminate the problem.

For stress incontinence, crossing your legs when you feel something like a sneeze coming on may prevent urine from leaking.

Pelvic floor exercises. These exercises, called Kegel exercises, involve squeezing and relaxing muscles in the pelvic and genital area. They strengthen your urinary sphincter and other muscles that control urination. Your doctor may

Performing Kegel exercises

One way to make sure you know how to contract your pelvic floor muscles is to try stopping the flow of urine while you're going to the bathroom. If you succeed, you already know the basics. A cautionary note: Don't continue to stop your urine stream. Doing Kegel exercises with a full bladder or while emptying your bladder can actually weaken the muscles. If you're having trouble finding the right muscles, don't be embarrassed to ask your doctor to help you learn to do the exercise correctly.

Once you've identified your pelvic floor muscles, empty your bladder and get into a sitting or standing position. Then firmly tense the muscles. Initially, you'll be instructed to keep the muscles contracted for 10 seconds, and relax them for 60 seconds between contractions. Complete a cycle of six sets (contracting, then relaxing) of Kegel exercises.

Be careful not to flex the muscles in your abdomen, thighs or buttocks. Also, try not to hold your breath. Just relax, breathe freely and focus on tightening only the pelvic floor muscles. Some men find it helpful to do the exercises while sitting on the toilet seat. It's recommended that you do them before bedtime with an empty bladder. This allows your muscles to rest afterwards, while you sleep.

Try to make it a habit to regularly perform the cycle of six sets of Kegel exercise at bedtime. The exercises will get easier the more often you do them. Later, you may also include a set while you do routine tasks, for example, as you commute to work. You can also vary your technique. Try doing sets of mini-Kegels — count quickly to 10 or 20, contracting and relaxing the pelvic floor muscles every time you say a number. Your health care team can advise you on additional exercise recommendations.

recommend that you do these exercises regularly to treat incontinence (For more on these exercises, see "Performing Kegel exercises" on page 168).

With Kegels, it can be difficult to know at first whether you're contracting the right muscles and in the right manner. In general, you'll sense a pulling-up feeling when you squeeze. Men may feel their penises pull in slightly toward their bodies.

After several months of doing these exercises correctly, muscle strength should gradually improve and you'll gain greater control. Kegel exercises are the most effective treatment for mild to moderate incontinence.

Medications. Many times, urinary incontinence can be corrected with the help of medication. Often, these medications are used in combination with behavior techniques.

Drugs commonly used to treat incontinence include anticholinergic (antispasmodic) drugs that help relax muscles and calm an overactive bladder. This class of drugs includes darifenacin (Enablex), oxybutynin (Ditropan), solifenacin (Vesicare), trospium (Sanctura) and tolterodine (Detrol).

Side effects of anticholinergic drugs may include dry mouth, blurred vision and constipation. To combat dry mouth, you may be tempted to drink more water, but this will affect your incontinence. Your doctor may recommend sucking on a piece of candy or chewing gum to produce more saliva.

You may also want to try an extended-release form of oxybutynin or tolterodine, or an oxybutynin skin patch. These forms of medication may have fewer side effects than the standard forms do.

Imipramine (Tofranil) is an antidepressant that may occasionally be used in combination with other medications to treat incontinence. This drug causes bladder muscles to relax and the urinary sphincter to contract.

If your incontinence is due to a urinary tract infection or an inflamed prostate, your doctor can successfully treat the problem with antibiotics.

Surgery. If other treatments aren't working and you continue to have leakage problems for at least a year without signs of improvement, your doctor may suggest surgery. Procedures that could help include:

Bulking material injections. The least invasive surgical procedure involves injecting a bulking substance into the lining of your urethra at the base of your bladder. The most common bulking agent is collagen, a protein found naturally in your body — but the agent for this procedure comes from cows.

An injection tightens the seal of the urinary sphincter by bulking up the surrounding tissue. The procedure is done with minimal anesthesia and typically takes about two to three minutes. You may need three or four injections before you notice an improvement in bladder control. And because your body absorbs the collagen, you'll probably need repeated injections.

If your incontinence is a result of radiation therapy, you may not be a good candidate for this procedure, because scar tissue caused by the radiation may prevent the bulking agent from working properly.

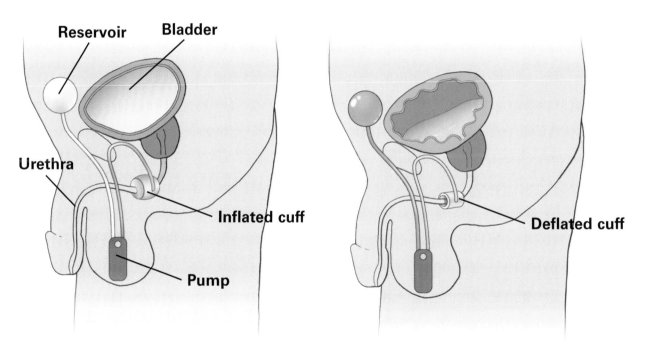

Artificial sphincter

An artificial sphincter uses a tiny silicone cuff placed around the urethra to treat incontinence. When inflated (left), the cuff squeezes the urethra, preventing urine from leaking. To urinate (right), you deflate the cuff, allowing urine to pass.

Artificial sphincter. This treatment involves a small, inflatable silicone cuff — the artificial sphincter — that's implanted around your urethra or the base of your bladder. The device operates like an arm cuff for taking blood pressure. When filled, it keeps the urethra closed until you're ready to urinate. It's particularly helpful for resolving severe, long-term incontinence.

The artificial sphincter inflates with fluid that's stored in a tiny reservoir in your lower abdomen. You inflate the cuff by triggering a pump implanted in your scrotum. The cuff squeezes the urethra shut, preventing urine flow. When you want to urinate, you press the same valve to deflate the cuff, allowing urine to flow out of your bladder.

Although total continence is not always achieved, this treatment is successful most of the time. Most people remain in the hospital for a few days after surgery. You can't use the sphincter for about six weeks, until your urethra and bladder have healed.

Sacral nerve stimulator. A stimulator, which resembles a pacemaker, is implanted under the skin in your abdomen. A wire from the device is connected to a sacral nerve, which runs through the spinal cord to your bladder. The device sends electric impulses that stimulate the nerve and help control bladder contractions.

Other procedures. Sometimes it's necessary to surgically remove blockages in your urinary tract, improve the position of your bladder neck or add support to weakened pelvic muscles.

Catheters and absorbent pads. Using catheters and absorbent pads doesn't eliminate incontinence but does ease the discomfort and inconvenience of leaking urine. They can be helpful when other treatments fail or while you're waiting for a treatment to take effect.

If you're incontinent because your bladder doesn't empty properly, your doctor may recommend that you learn how to insert a thin, flexible tube (catheter) into your urethra several times a day to drain your bladder. In certain circumstances, the catheter may be left in. The catheter is connected to a small, external bag to hold urine. As needed, the bag is emptied.

Catheterization should give you more control over leakage, especially if you have overflow incontinence. Although the procedure sounds difficult and painful, after a few times most men lose their anxiety and are comfortable performing it.

An alternative option may be the use of an external catheter, which fits over the penis. Urine is collected in a bag that must be regularly emptied.

If you aren't using a catheter or the catheter is removed, you may need absorbent pads or protective garments to help manage urine loss. Most products are no more bulky than normal underwear and you can wear them easily under everyday clothing. Other products are heavily padded and designed to be worn only at home or during the night.

Men who have problems with dribbles of urine can use a drip collector — a small pocket of absorbent padding that's worn over the penis and held in place by closefitting underwear. Men can also wear panty liners or pads of varying thickness inside regular cloth underwear. These products may be purchased at drugstores, supermarkets and medical supply stores.

Penile clamps. This device fits over your penis, and its tightness can be adjusted to stop the flow of urine.

However, it should not be worn for more than two to three hours at a time. If left on for too long, it can cause tissue damage, swelling and pain.

Treating erectile dysfunction

Erectile dysfunction (ED) is the inability of a man to maintain a firm erection long enough to have sex. Sometimes called impotence, ED was once considered a psychological issue or natural consequence of growing older. It's now known that erectile dysfunction is more often a disruption of a complex physical process involving your brain, hormones, nerves, muscles and blood vessels.

Erectile dysfunction can be a result of your prostate cancer or its treatment. As the cancer grows, it can invade and damage the nerves attached to your prostate gland that control erections. Cancer treatment such as surgery, radiation and cryotherapy also can damage these nerves.

Although the use of hormone therapy to treat prostate cancer doesn't injure the nerves physically, it almost completely eliminates testosterone, leaving you with no desire for sexual activity. The nerves still function, but nothing stimulates them.

Although you may view erectile dysfunction as a personal and embarrassing problem, it's important that you seek treatment. In most cases, ED can be successfully treated.

The cause and severity of your ED helps determine which is the best treatment or combination of treatments. Cost also may be a consideration, since insurance coverage may vary for options such as medications.

Medication

For treating erectile dysfunction, most doctors turn first to one of the following types of prescription drugs.

Oral medications. Medications in tablet or capsule form that are available to treat ED include:
- Sildenafil (Viagra)
- Tadalafil (Cialis)
- Vardenafil (Levitra)

All three medications work in much the same way. Chemically known as phosphodiesterase inhibitors, these drugs enhance the effects of nitric oxide, a chemical that relaxes muscles in the penis. This increases the amount of blood flow and allows a natural erection sequence to take place.

These medications don't automatically produce an erection. You'll still require sexual stimulation — physical and emotional — for the erection to occur. Regardless of the situation, many men experience improvement in erectile function after this treatment.

These medications share many similarities, but they have differences as well. They vary in dosage, the duration of effectiveness and possible side effects. Your doctor will help you decide the best time to take a medication before sexual activity. None should be taken more than once every 24 hours.

Other differences — for example, which drug may be best suited for certain types of men — aren't yet known. No rigorous study has directly compared all the three medications.

Consult your doctor to find the best type of drug for you. Individual dosages may need adjusting. Or you may need to alter your schedule to take the medication. Your doctor will probably start you on an average dose and increase or decrease the amount you take, depending on your individual response to the medication.

Not all men can or should take these medications to treat erectile dysfunction. Avoid these medications if:

- You take nitrate drugs for angina, such as nitroglycerin (Nitro-Bid, others), isosorbide mononitrate (Imdur) and isosorbide dinitrate (Isordil)
- You take certain types of alpha blockers for an enlarged prostate or for high blood pressure

In addition, these drugs may not be a good choice if you have metabolic risk factors such as severe heart disease, heart failure, stroke, very low blood pressure, uncontrolled high blood pressure or uncontrolled diabetes.

Sildenafil, tadalafil and vardenafil may cause side effects, including facial flushing, which generally lasts no more than five to 10 minutes. You might also experience mild headache, upset stomach, muscle aches and heartburn. Higher doses can produce short-term visual problems, including blurred vision and increased light sensitivity, as well as hearing problems, ringing in

the ears and dizziness. These effects generally subside a few hours after taking the drug.

Alprostadil. Two different treatments involve the drug alprostadil, which is a synthetic version of the natural hormone prostaglandin E. The medication helps relax muscle tissue in the penis, which increases the blood flow needed for an erection.

Sometimes, alprostadil is combined with other types of medication to

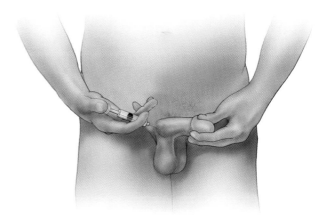

Needle-injection therapy

Self-injection introduces the drug alprostadil directly to the penis to increase blood flow and cause an erection. It takes several minutes to take effect.

improve its effects. Instead of being taken as a pill, alprostadil is delivered in one of two ways:

Needle-injection therapy. With this treatment, you use a fine needle to inject alprostadil (Caverject) at the base of your penis. The medication needs to go into one of the two cylindrical, sponge-like structures that run along the length of your penis on each side — these structures fill with blood when they're stimulated.

It generally takes five to 20 minutes for the drug to take effect, and the erection usually lasts from about 40 to 60 minutes. Because the needle is very thin — like needles used for diabetes and allergies — pain from the injection is usually minor.

You'll need to be careful to inject the needle on the side of your penis and not at the top or the bottom. Located on top are arteries, veins and nerves, and on the bottom is the urethra. If you hit either of these areas with the needle, you won't get an erection and you'll need to wait at least 24 hours before you can use the medication again. If a misplaced injection happens more than once, contact your doctor for more instruction.

Side effects may include bleeding from the injection, and on rare occasions, a prolonged, painful erection (priapism).

To minimize the risk of prolonged erection, it's important that you test the medication to determine the proper dose. If an erection continues for more than four hours, the blood trapped inside your penis becomes thick because of oxygen loss, which can damage your penis.

Call your doctor or go to an emergency room if the erection continues for more than four hours. Next time, you may need to decrease the amount of medication in order to reduce the duration of the erection.

Other side effects, which also are rare, may include a lump (fibrosis) where you inject the drug. It usually goes away when you stop the injections. Ways to prevent fibrosis are to vary the injection site and to limit the injections to two or three times a week.

Self-administered intraurethral therapy. This method uses a disposable applicator to insert a tiny alprostadil suppository — about half the size of a grain of rice — into the tip of your penis. The drug is delivered as the suppository dissolves. The brand name of this suppository is Muse.

The suppository, placed about 2 inches into your urethra, is absorbed by the erectile tissue in your penis, increasing the blood flow that causes an erection. It generally takes about 10 minutes for the medication to take effect.

A rubber ring placed around the base of your penis before the suppository is inserted helps trap blood and maintain an erection. Each pellet is good for one application.

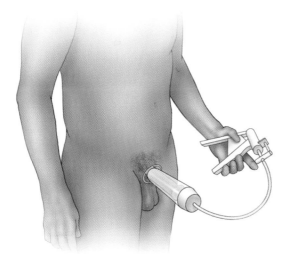

Vacuum erection device

This device uses a hand pump to draw blood into the penis and create an erection. An elastic ring placed at the base of the penis keeps it erect.

Side effects may include some pain, dizziness and formation of hard, fibrous tissue. After a test dose in the doctor's office, you can learn to do the procedure yourself.

Vacuum erection devices

These devices use vacuum pressure to draw blood into your penis. You place an airtight, plastic tube over your penis, attached to a hand-powered or battery-powered pump. By using the pump, you draw air out of the plastic tube. This creates a vacuum effect, which pulls blood into the tissue of your penis. The increased blood flow produces an erection.

When you achieve an adequate erection from the pump, you slip an elastic ring around the base of your penis. The ring traps the blood inside your penis, allowing you to keep the erection once the tube is removed. Remove the ring within 30 minutes to restore normal blood flow. If you don't, you could damage penile tissue.

Some men find the elastic ring uncomfortable and believe that it looks unnatural. In addition, your penis may feel cold because there's no blood circulation. However, a vacuum pump works in most cases and doesn't require medication or surgery.

Penile implants

If other treatments fail or don't work well, another option to consider is having a surgical implant. This treatment involves surgically placed devices on both sides of the penis that help support it. This will allow an erection to occur for as often and as long as you desire. Currently, there are two types of penile implants in use:

- *Semirigid, bendable implant.* This is the easiest implant to use and the least likely to malfunction. Two hard, but flexible, rods give you a permanent erection. You bend your penis down toward your body to hide the erection, and bend it up to have sexual intercourse.

- *Inflatable implant with pump.* Two hollow cylinders implanted into your penis are connected to a tiny pump in your scrotum. When you squeeze the pump, fluid from an implanted reservoir fills the cylinders and produces an erection. Instead of having a permanent erection, you produce an erection only when you want one.

Relieving bowel disorders

Some men who receive radiation therapy for prostate cancer experience a variety of gastrointestinal complications. These may include blood in the stool, cramps, rectal irritation and discharge, diarrhea, and a feeling of urinary urgency. Generally, these complications are annoying and worrisome but temporary.

External beam radiotherapy is very accurate in targeting prostate cancer, but your rectum will also usually receive some of the radiation. The most common side effect is rectal irritation. This irritation should lessen once treatment is completed but sometimes it can persist. Injury from radiation that requires surgical repair is rare.

Prostate surgery also can cause rectal injury. However, this result also is rare. Often, if there's an injury, it's usually repaired during the actual surgery with no permanent damage.

The bowel disorders may continue for several months after prostate treatment. Most improve on their own.

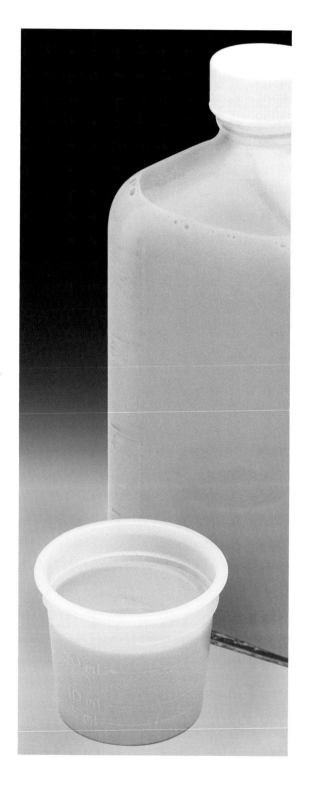

Blood in the stool

Radiation therapy may injure the lining of your rectum. One result may be the abnormal growth of tiny blood vessels (capillaries) near the surface. These capillaries have thin, fragile walls that tear or rupture easily. Sometimes, rectal bleeding can continue for years.

Treatment depends on the severity of the bleeding. Often, the first step is to monitor the bleeding to see if you're passing only small amounts of blood. If the bleeding is moderate to heavy, your doctor may prescribe stool softeners or medicated enemas to reduce pressure on your rectal lining as the stool passes. For severe cases, laser therapy can often destroy or seal off the blood vessels that cause the bleeding.

Diarrhea

Diarrhea may result from radiation therapy, but usually only when it's necessary to treat the entire pelvic region. Signs and symptoms include frequent, loose, watery stools, abdominal cramps and pain, and bloating. Generally, the effects are temporary. Over-the-counter anti-diarrheal medications such as Imodium, Kaopectate or Pepto-Bismol may help reduce your symptoms.

Diarrhea may cause the loss of significant amounts of water and salts. To prevent dehydration during episodes of diarrhea, drink at least eight glasses of clear liquids a day, including water or clear sodas. Avoid dairy products, caffeine, and fatty or highly seasoned foods, which can prolong diarrhea. Signs of dehydration include excessive thirst, dry mouth, weakness, dark-colored urine, and little or no urination.

Constipation

Medications to treat prostate cancer may reduce the normal activity of your bowels and delay bowel movements. When this happens, fecal material becomes packed and hard, producing cramps and constipation.

Signs and symptoms of constipation include passing hard stools, straining frequently during bowel movements, and experiencing bloating and abdominal discomfort.

Fortunately, you may be able to relieve constipation by following a regular eating schedule and including high-fiber foods, such as whole-grain cereals and breads, fresh vegetables, and fresh fruits. Add these foods to your diet gradually to avoid possible discomfort caused by gas. Exercising daily and drinking plenty of fluids also will help reduce constipation.

You may also try a natural fiber supplement, such as Citrucel, Fiberall or Metamucil, which should help within one to three days. Fiber supplements are generally safe, but are also very absorbent — so be sure to drink plenty of water or other fluids. Otherwise, fiber supplements can actually become constipating — the opposite of what you want them to do.

If these measures don't help, ask your doctor about using a stool softener or laxative. There are several types:

Stool softeners. These are the most gentle products. They're sold over-the-counter under a variety of brand names, including Colace, Correctol and Surfak. Mineral oil shouldn't be taken as a stool softener because it can block the absorption of key vitamins. In general, you shouldn't rely on stool softeners on a regular basis because they can cause other problems.

Saline laxatives. These include the over-the-counter product Phillips' Milk of Magnesia, which works by increasing water content in your stool.

Stimulant laxatives. These are more powerful products and should be taken only when other measures fail to induce a bowel movement. Over-the-counter brand names include Dulcolax, Ex-Lax and Senokot.

Answers to your questions

How long should I expect to wear absorbent underwear after treatment for prostate cancer?

The length of time varies. One to four months isn't unusual.

What's the difference between impotence and erectile dysfunction?

The terms are often used interchangeably, but they aren't exactly the same. Impotence means that your penis is unable to become firm (erect) or stay firm long enough to have sexual intercourse. Erectile dysfunction includes impotence, plus other abnormalities, such as prolonged erection or abnormal curvature of the penis.

If I have good erections before treatment, does that increase the chance I'll be able to have normal erections afterward?

Yes. Younger, healthier men experiencing strong erections are far more likely to continue normal erections after treatment than are older men or men already having erectile problems.

Are treatments for incontinence and erectile dysfunction covered by Medicare?

Most are. However, Medicare may not pay the entire cost, especially for medications. You may have to pay a portion of the cost yourself.

Chapter 10

Getting on with life

Receiving a diagnosis of prostate cancer may have been one of the most difficult challenges you ever faced. The diagnosis may have consumed your thoughts and actions and produced many long-lasting changes to your daily routines, relationships with others and outlook on life.

As treatment started, you may have struggled to retain any sense of normalcy. You likely experienced a range of emotions, including disbelief, anger, anxiety, emptiness and depression. You may be facing side effects of treatment that are both discomforting and emotionally difficult to accept. You've probably felt an ongoing need to rethink your life expectations and reprioritize your goals.

Now with the course of treatment well under way, you may be wondering what more the future has in store for you — what will your quality of life be like? What long-term outcomes can you hope to expect?

Although prostate cancer remains a serious illness, it's no longer considered an inevitable death sentence. Knowledge of the cancer — its effect on your body, how to detect it and how best to treat it — has come a long way. Increasingly, prostate cancer is becoming a tale of survivorship.

You can learn to cope with the impact of this disease. Life with and after prostate cancer not only is possible but also can be fulfilling.

Medical visits

Some men dread visiting their doctor following treatment for prostate cancer. This is natural — a routine doctor visit is probably how they first became aware of this life-changing development. Even follow-up care can cause feelings of anxiety, stress and sadness, often because of a fear of recurrence.

Try to balance your anxiety with positive thoughts. Keep in mind that the treatment you've received, and will continue to receive, helps you. Ask your doctor when you have questions, such as how frequently you'll need checkups and what tests you'll receive.

At first, you may need to see your doctor every three months. Eventually, your visits may be just once or twice a

Talking to your doctor

If you have questions about what to expect after treatment for prostate cancer, discuss them with your doctor. Here are 10 questions to get you started:

1. "How often will I need a checkup?"
2. "What will my checkups consist of, and will they always be the same?"
3. "What are some signs that my cancer has returned or progressed?"
4. "How likely are these signs or symptoms to occur?"
5. "What changes might I see that are OK — that aren't danger signs?"
6. "Should I change my diet?"
7. "Do I need to alter my daily routine?"
8. "If I experience pain, what should I do?"
9. "What's the best way for me to get in touch with you if I have questions?"
10. "Is there someone else I can talk to if you aren't available?"

Adapted from "Facing Forward: A Guide for Cancer Survivors," National Cancer Institute, National Institutes of Health, 2002

year. In addition to a physical exam, each checkup may include X-rays and a prostate-specific antigen (PSA) test to help determine whether the cancer has returned or progressed.

Emotional toll

Prostate cancer can produce a roller coaster of emotions. But there's no "right way" to feel or act if you have cancer. Feelings are simply feelings — they aren't right or wrong. It's what you do with those feelings — recognizing and dealing with them instead of bottling them up — that's most important.

What to expect

Certain feelings and emotions seem to be more common than are others in people coping with prostate cancer. You may experience all of them, just a few of them or none of them.

Anxiety. The distress caused by your diagnosis and treatment or just living with cancer can lead to anxiety. You may be anxious about tests and procedures, changes to your body, loss of control, a cancer recurrence or death. These feelings are normal.

If you experience side effects from your treatment, such as incontinence or erectile dysfunction, talking about them may embarrass you. These side effects can also undermine self-confidence. You may withdraw from social gatherings because you're afraid of embarrassing yourself.

The signs and symptoms of anxiety include:
- Intense fear or worry
- Restlessness or irritability
- Trouble sleeping or waking up feeling wired
- Fatigue or loss of energy
- Impaired concentration
- Rapid pulse, shortness of breath and trembling

A good relationship with your doctor can help you deal with some of the fears and concerns that fuel anxiety. Family and friends also can provide support by helping to reduce the amount of stress in your life.

Usually, anxiety tends to dissipate as you adjust to the changes you're going through. But sometimes these feelings persist. Anxiety is treatable, and addressing it promptly can enhance your well-being and make your cancer less worrisome.

Depression. Depression is common among people with cancer. You may grow discouraged and deeply pessimistic about your future. Although these feelings take time to work through, they usually become more manageable over weeks or months.

Among some people, these feelings deepen and linger. Grief and discouragement can evolve into major depression. This can precipitate a downward spiral that makes you more miserable. Because you're depressed, you don't put effort into coping with your daily problems. And when the problems get worse, so does your depression.

Major depression is characterized by a change in mood that lasts for more than two weeks. Signs and symptoms of depression include:

- Persistent anger or sadness
- Irritability or feelings of anxiety
- Lack of interest in most activities
- Noticeable changes in appetite and sleep patterns
- Fatigue or loss of energy
- Feelings of helplessness, hopelessness, worthlessness or guilt
- Continuous negative thinking
- Impaired concentration
- Recurrent thoughts of death or suicide

Depression is a serious health problem — it's not a passing phase that goes away on its own. When left untreated, the symptoms of depression tend to get worse. And the condition is not something you can handle on your own — it must be professionally treated. Learn to recognize the symptoms of depression and immediately consult your doctor when you feel that depression could be developing.

Similar to anxiety, treatment for depression usually involves a combination of medications and therapy sessions with a psychiatrist or counselor. Most people who seek treatment show improvement within a matter of weeks.

If you're in the midst of active cancer treatment, eliminating depression can help you better cope with your cancer therapy and any side effects it may have. It will also improve your relationships with family and friends.

Sense of loss. After surgery to remove your prostate, you may feel an emptiness that's hard to describe, especially if the surgery causes erectile dysfunction. Treatment often reduces or eliminates the production of male hormones, mainly testosterone — which can affect how you respond to sexual stimulation.

Because of these side effects, you might sense that you're somehow less of a man — just as some women may feel they're less feminine after breast removal. Fortunately, many treatments for erectile dysfunction are available that can help ease these concerns.

What you can do

As you learn to cope with the changes in your life, strong emotions should become more manageable. Many people are surprised to discover reserves of strength they never thought they had. But years later, you may have times when you struggle to conquer feelings of anxiety or discouragement related to your cancer. This is normal. What's important is that the balance of your emotions leans to the positive side.

The following strategies may help you cope with some of the residual effects of prostate cancer:

Be prepared. Educating yourself about the illness and the available treatment options can help you feel more in control of your life. Write down questions and concerns and bring them with you to doctor visits. Often, the fewer surprises you face, the more quickly you can adapt. But don't let your quest for knowledge become an obsession, which may cause you more stress or to second-guess your doctor.

Maintain a normal routine. Don't let the cancer or the side effects of treatment control your life. Try to maintain a semblance of your former lifestyle and daily routine. You'll do better if you can engage in activities that give you a sense of purpose, fulfillment and meaning — return to work, take a trip or join a family outing. If you have health limitations, give yourself permission to start slowly and gradually build your level of endurance.

Build a positive support system. Your mind and body aren't separate. The better you feel emotionally, the better able you'll be to physically cope with cancer. Surrounding yourself with caring people who support you will boost your spirits and give you confidence.

Take care of your body. Get enough sleep, eat a healthy diet and exercise regularly, as you're able to. Exercise helps release tension in muscles and reduces stress. It's been shown to decrease depressive signs and symptoms, improve negative mood, increase self-esteem, and have a positive effect on your quality of life.

Spirituality and healing

Spiritual peace can be a powerful healing force. Spirituality is often confused with religion. But spirituality isn't so much connected to a specific belief or form of worship as it is with the spirit or the soul. Spirituality is about meaning, values and purpose in life.

Religion may be one way of expressing spirituality, but it's not the only way. For some people, spirituality is feeling in tune with nature and the universe. For others, spirituality is expressed through music, meditation or art.

Numerous studies have attempted to measure the effect of spirituality on illness and recovery. Many researchers believe that people who consider themselves to be spiritual enjoy better health, live longer, recover from illness more quickly and with fewer complications, have less depression and chemical addiction, have lower blood pressure, and cope better with serious disease, including cancer.

No one knows exactly how spirituality affects health. Some experts attribute the healing effect to hope, which is known to benefit your immune system. Others liken spiritual acts and beliefs to meditation, which decreases muscle tension and can lower your heart rate. Still others point to the social connectedness that spirituality often provides.

An important point to keep in mind is that although spirituality is associated with healing and better health, it isn't a cure. Spirituality can help you live more fully despite your symptoms, but no studies have found that it actually cures health problems. It's best to view spirituality as a helpful healing force — as a supplement to, but not a substitute for, traditional medical care.

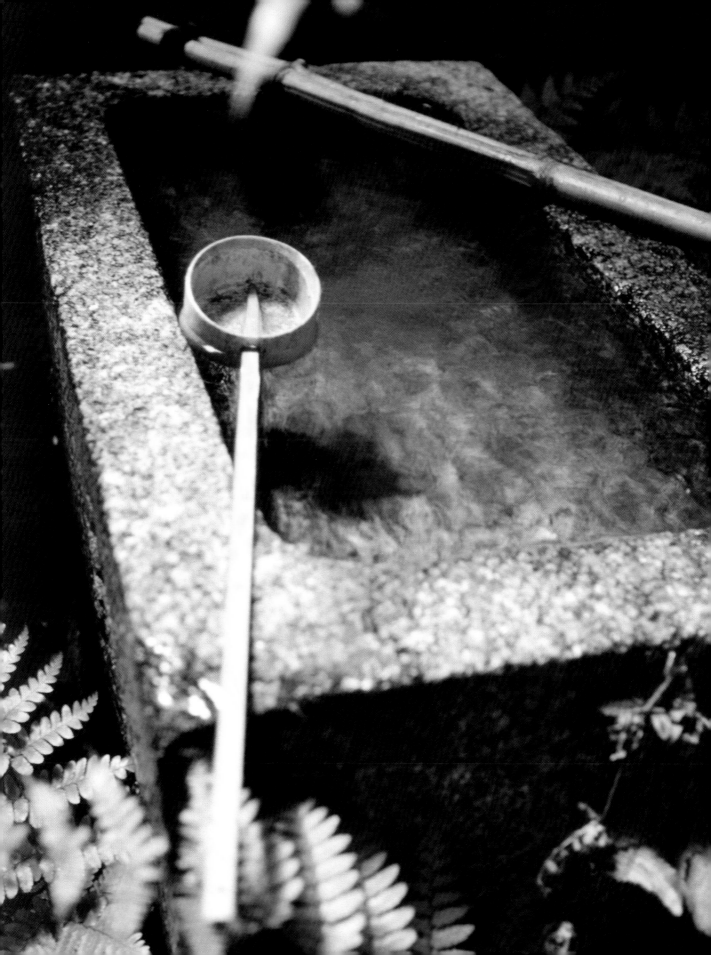

Simple ways to relax

Wrestling with heavy emotions, such as anxiety and depression, can contribute to fatigue. Relaxation helps relieve stress that makes it difficult for you to concentrate and recuperate. Talk to your doctor about stress-reduction techniques, and which ones might work best for you.

Deep breathing. Breathing from your diaphragm is more relaxing than is breathing from your chest. It exchanges more carbon dioxide for oxygen, giving you more energy.

Progressive muscle relaxation. This technique involves relaxing a series of muscles one at a time. First, raise the tension level in a group of muscles, such as a leg or arm, by tightening the muscles and then slowly relaxing them. Concentrate on letting the tension go in each muscle. Then move on to the next muscle group.

Word repetition. Choose a word or phrase that's a cue for you to relax, and then constantly repeat it. While repeating the word or phrase, try to breathe deeply and slowly and think of something that gives you pleasant sensations of warmth and heaviness.

Guided imagery. Lie quietly and picture yourself in a pleasant and peaceful setting. Experience the setting with all of your senses, as if you were actually there. For instance, imagine lying on a beach. Picture the beautiful blue sky, smell the salt water, hear the waves, and feel the warm breeze on your skin. The messages your brain gets help calm and relax you.

Find ways to compensate for side effects. For example, if you have problems with incontinence, sit at the back of the movie theater or meeting room instead of the front. That way you'll be nearer to a bathroom if you need one. Similarly, sit in an aisle seat on airplanes, trains or buses. Wear absorbent undergarments if you're not sure whether you'll be near a bathroom. Avoid caffeinated products and alcohol because they increase urination.

Don't avoid sexual contact. Your natural reaction to erectile dysfunction may be to avoid all sexual contact. Don't fall for this course of action — there are many ways to express your sexuality. Touching, holding, hugging and caressing may become far more important to you and your partner. In fact, the closeness you develop in these actions can produce greater sexual intimacy than you've ever had before.

Look for the silver lining. Cancer doesn't have to be all negative — good can come out of your experience. Confrontation with cancer may lead you to grow emotionally and spiritually, identify what really matters to you, settle long-standing disputes, and spend more time with the people who are important to you.

Regaining your strength

Fatigue is one of the most common side effects of prostate cancer. In part, fatigue is a reaction to the physical and emotional toll that the cancer takes.

For someone who hasn't experienced cancer-related fatigue, it can be difficult to grasp what it's like. Everyone knows what it feels like to run out of steam after a hectic day, but a little rest usually helps you bounce back. Cancer-related fatigue is more pervasive, and rest may not make it better.

Fatigue may result from:
- Stress and depression
- Sleep disturbances
- Surgery or radiation therapy
- Metabolic abnormalities related to the cancer or its treatment
- Low red blood cell count (anemia) from the cancer or its treatment

Other factors that may contribute to your fatigue include medications, poor nutrition and lack of activity. If you're experiencing cancer-related fatigue, consult with a member of your health care team for help.

Self-care for fatigue

Ignoring exhaustion and pushing yourself too hard may make your fatigue worse. At the same time, resting or sleeping more doesn't cure fatigue. Find help from your social network.

Many people value their independence, and asking others for help is a new and unwanted experience. But it's important to accept that you can't do it all. Call on friends and family to help with chores and errands.

Other steps that may help you reduce fatigue include:

- Plan activities for times when you have the most energy.
- Look for ways to conserve energy. For example, sit on a stool when you're in the workshop or kitchen.
- Delegate chores. You may need to ask others to help you with tasks that you've always done before. But don't use your illness as an excuse to avoid all chores — some physical activity is good.
- Pace yourself. Take short naps or rest breaks when you need them.
- Establish an exercise program to help lessen your fatigue. Moderate exercise after cancer treatment is strongly recommended.

- Eat a good breakfast to prepare your body for the day's demands. Then refuel every three or four hours.
- Make sure you're drinking enough fluids. Dehydration can contribute to fatigue.
- Tell your doctor if fatigue remains a problem. There may be a physical cause that can be treated.

Get a good night's sleep. Fatigue often interferes with sleep. Here are suggestions that can help you sleep better:

- Get in the habit of going to bed and waking up at about the same times each day. This helps your body establish a regular sleep cycle.
- Develop a nightly routine before getting into bed — perhaps it's reading, bathing or relaxing in front of the television. This signals your body to prepare for sleep.
- Avoid foods and beverages that can disrupt sleep. Anything with caffeine, such as coffee or chocolate, can make it more difficult to fall asleep. Alcoholic drinks may help you fall asleep but can disrupt deep-sleep patterns.
- Getting at least 30 minutes of physical activity daily — preferably five to six hours before you go to bed — and keeping active during the day helps you to sleep better at night.

Fear of recurrence

One of the most common fears among prostate cancer survivors is that the cancer will come back. While it's true that cancer can recur after treatment, it's also true that many men never experience a recurrence.

But we live in a world that emphasizes facts and knowledge. Despite certain clues about the general outcome of prostate cancer and cancer treatment, it's impossible to foretell the future. Therefore, you and your doctor must learn to live with some degree of uncertainty.

Some anxiety about recurrence is healthy — for example, it prompts you to respond to unusual signs and symptoms. Being continuously anxious, however, can rob you of time that might be spent in a more worthwhile manner, such as focusing on work or family or simply enjoying life.

- Block out noise, either by closing your door or creating subtle background noise with a fan. Keep your bedroom temperature comfortable, and drink fewer beverages before bed so that you won't have to get up as often during the night.

The amount of sleep needed each night varies from person to person, but the average is around eight hours.

Eating better to feel better

Food provides the fuel that allows your body to maintain its strength and function best. A nutritious diet is especially important when your body is undergoing the rigors of cancer treatment.

The problem is that cancer treatment may cause nausea and vomiting, and may affect your appetite. Food may not taste the way it used to before you started treatments. You may have difficulty swallowing, or your mouth may become dry.

When you're being treated for cancer, what you eat and how often you eat may be different from when you're healthy. Normally, good nutrition stresses fruits, vegetables and grains, and cutting back on fat and sugar. For people undergoing cancer treatment, a lack of appetite can make this difficult.

If you don't eat enough food or the right kinds of foods, your body resorts to using nutrients that have been stored in cells. Drawing on these reserves may weaken your natural defenses against infection. To prevent this, try to eat high-calorie foods that promote energy. Also, eat adequate protein-containing foods that give you strength and help repair body tissues.

The better you eat, the more able you may be to handle chemotherapy or radiation treatments. The following tips may help you make every bite count.

Increase calories. During cancer treatment, your need for calories is often greater than usual. Maintaining your weight is a helpful sign that you're eating enough. You can add calories by:

- Using butter, margarine, mayonnaise, oil, cream cheese, gravies, sauces, salad dressings, sour cream, and other fatty spreads or toppings. Sauteed or fried foods are higher in calories than are baked, broiled or steamed items.
- Topping foods with sugar, jam, jelly and honey. Sweetened cereals and granola and sweetened fresh or canned fruit and juices are higher in calories than are their unsweetened counterparts.
- Peanut butter, nuts, dried fruit and ice cream are calorie-packed snacks.
- Drinking beverages with calories — fruit juices, lemonade, soft drinks and fortified fruit drinks. Add sugar or cream to coffee and tea.

Maintain protein intake. Eating adequate amounts of protein doesn't necessarily mean eating large amounts of meat. Other options include:

- About 2 to 3 ounces of poultry, fish or shellfish at meals. Think of these foods as condiments rather than a main course. Include them in pasta dishes, casseroles and stir-fries.
- Foods such as beans and tofu that are high in protein and can substitute for meat. The soy in tofu may make cancer cells more vulnerable to radiation.
- Eggs — fried, scrambled or hard-boiled — can make a healthy meal. Eggs can also be used in custards, sandwich fillings and French toast.
- Cheese served with crackers, added to sandwiches, or melted onto vegetables. A half cup of cottage cheese with fruit is a healthy snack.
- Milk and milk products. Because of the possible role of calcium in prostate cancer, try to keep milk and yogurt consumption to no more than 2 cups daily to help ensure adequate protein intake.

Stock up on nutritional drinks. These products, commonly available as a liquid or powder, are sold under brand names such as Ensure, Sustacal, Boost and Carnation Instant Breakfast. The

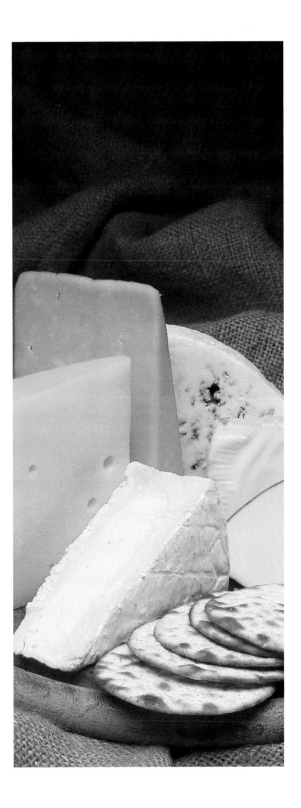

Curbing nausea and diarrhea

Radiation, medications and anxiety all may contribute to nausea and diarrhea. Here are practical suggestions to help you combat these conditions:

Nausea
- Eat mild-flavored, nonfatty foods such as cereals, rice, noodles, baked potatoes, lean meats, fish, chicken, cottage cheese, fruits and vegetables.
- Eat something dry, such as a piece of toast or saltine crackers, right after you wake up in the morning.
- Foods that are cool or at room temperature may be more appealing because they produce less odor than do hot foods.
- Avoid foods that are overly sweet, fried, spicy or fatty because they're more likely to trigger nausea.
- After you've eaten, sit up for 10 to 20 minutes and let your food settle.

Diarrhea
- Drink plenty of clear fluids, and eat food in small amounts throughout the day instead of three large meals.
- Avoid greasy foods, foods with skins or seeds, and gas-forming vegetables, such as broccoli, cabbage and cauliflower.
- Eat foods and drink liquids that contain potassium and sodium — two minerals often lost during diarrhea. High-sodium liquids include bouillon and broth. Foods and beverages high in potassium include bananas, peach or apricot nectar, and boiled or mashed potatoes. Sports drinks contain high levels of both sodium and potassium.

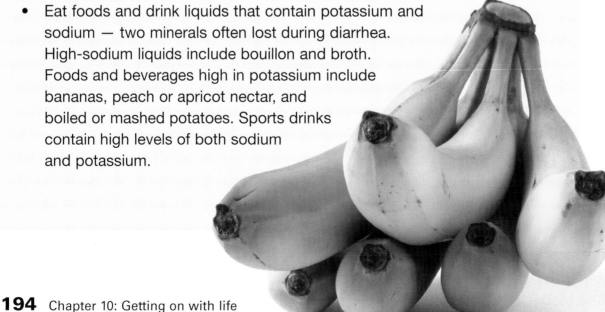

drinks are high in calories and protein, and contain extra vitamins and minerals.

Nutritional drinks can be used as meal substitutes if you don't feel like eating. You can also drink them between meals in order to improve your diet and increase calories, protein and other nutrients. Because the drinks need no refrigeration, you may carry them with you and have them whenever you feel hungry or thirsty.

Some people find nutritional products difficult to drink because they don't care for the flavor or texture. If this is true for you, try this simple recipe and see if it improves the product's appeal: Combine one can of a liquid drink with a piece of fruit or a scoop of ice cream. Blend the mixture in a blender and serve over ice.

Stimulating your appetite

The nausea that you may experience during chemotherapy can make food unappealing. To improve your diet and stimulate your appetite:

Eat lightly and frequently. Sticking to a three-meals-a-day schedule may be difficult when you're fighting cancer. If your appetite and taste buds seem in disarray, eating smaller meals throughout the day may work better — even if it's just a few bites every hour or so. Ordinarily, people shouldn't eat at bedtime but do so if you're up to it.

Prepare and freeze meals ahead of time. This allows you to have something quick and easy to fix on days when you don't feel like cooking.

Choose foods that look and smell good to you. Some cancer treatments can change your sense of taste and smell. So if red meat becomes unappetizing, for example, switch to other sources of protein such as chicken, fish, eggs or dairy products.

Most people being treated for cancer find soups and soft foods are the easiest to eat and digest. Lightly seasoned dishes made with eggs, poultry and pasta are generally well tolerated.

Be willing to try new foods. You may find that some foods you used to love now taste bad, making it even harder to eat enough. On the other hand, foods you used to avoid may now be more appealing. Give them a try.

Don't force yourself to eat favorite foods. Especially when you're nauseated, trying to eat favorite foods may leave you with a permanent distaste for these items — you may forever link them with the unpleasant side effects. Consider saving your favorite foods for when you're feeling better.

Enhance flavor. Try adding small amounts of seasoning if food tastes bland. You can also marinate poultry and meat in fruit juices, sweet wine — if permitted — or sauces.

Drink less with meals. Sufficient beverages are vital to good nutrition — aim for 6 to 8 cups of fluid daily. But try to limit beverages at mealtimes because they can make you feel full when you're not. Instead, save them for the end of the meal.

Change the atmosphere. Eating in a different setting may stimulate your appetite. Invite a friend over, play music, light some candles, or watch a favorite television program.

If you still have trouble eating a few weeks after your treatment, ask your doctor for advice. A registered dietitian who specializes in helping people with cancer can devise an eating plan that's better suited to your tastes and special nutritional needs.

Continuing to work

Having cancer doesn't mean that your career is finished, or you'll never again be able to pull your weight on the job. In fact, the vast majority of people with cancer do return to work. Surveys show that people who have been treated for cancer can be just as productive as other workers, and no more likely to take sick days.

Your job is an important part of your life, contributing to your personal fulfillment, self-image, income, enjoyment and sense of community. A job also has therapeutic value, providing a welcome distraction from your cancer. Many men with prostate cancer find that getting back to work helps them regain a sense of normalcy in their lives.

At first, you may need to make a few adjustments. Work can be exhausting if you try to do too much too soon. But eventually you should be able to resume your routine.

Under the Americans With Disabilities Act, your employer is required by law to make reasonable accommodations

Getting your life in order

A common response to a cancer diagnosis — even when the prognosis is good — is to reorganize your life. You may feel a need to review insurance policies, update your will, and clean out closets and basement, giving away items you no longer need.

This concern is understandable. Cancer makes you think about life — what's really important, what you want to achieve, and if you should die, how you can make things easier for your family. Planning for the future is good. It can save hardships and disagreements later on.

Be prepared that your family may view your actions with concern. They may feel you've lost all hope and that you're giving up. Take time to talk with family members about what you're doing. It may help alleviate their anxiety.

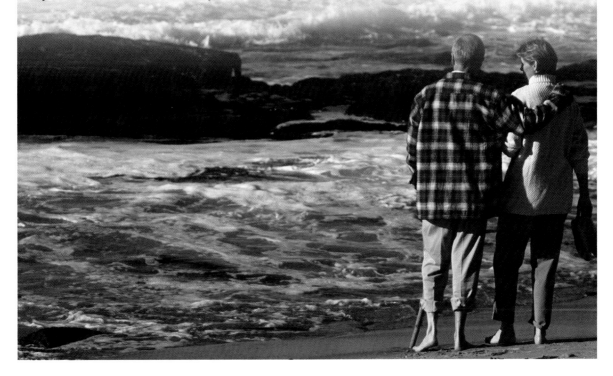

that enable you to work while you're undergoing treatment and recuperating. These laws may not apply to certain organizations, such as employers with fewer than 15 employees.

The accommodations your employer may provide include:
- Flexible work hours
- Work from home, if possible
- Use of earned sick and vacation leave with pay, in accordance with your company's policies
- Use of unpaid leave
- Moving your workstation to a better location

Discuss with your doctor about how to ease back into a work schedule. Talk to your supervisor to prepare for your return. Consider how you'll respond to co-workers who may have questions about how you're doing. Practicing what you'll say ahead of time can make the interchange more comfortable.

Communicating with others

Cancer has a way of stifling communication when you need it the most.

Family members may have difficulty coming to grips with your illness, which may prevent them from talking about the important issues.

Well-meaning friends — not knowing what to say or do, and not wanting to upset you — may steer clear of conversations about your health. Others may make inappropriate statements or ask more questions than you feel comfortable answering.

A period of adjustment may be necessary for everyone involved. Here are ways you can make it easier for others to adjust and provide support:

Accept the emotional timetables of everyone. You may want to talk about important issues related to your illness before some of your family and friends are ready. If they're not ready to talk, give them more time to adjust. Look for clues in their body language, for example, whether they make eye contact or not.

If a loved one is ready to talk before you are, postpone the discussion without hurting the person's feelings. Place responsibility on yourself by saying, "I know we need to make some decisions. But I really need a little more time."

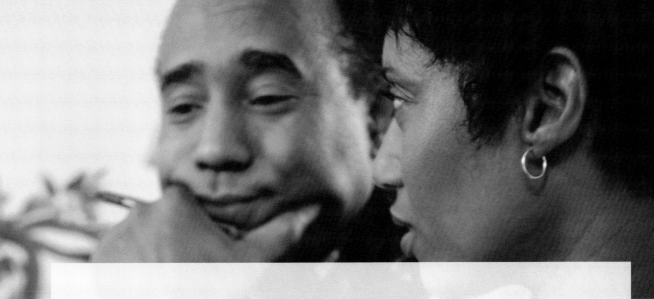

Coping with survival

Traditionally, a cancer survivor is someone in whom there's no evidence of active disease five years after treatment. Despite the relief of winning the battle, survival can bring other emotional challenges.

During cancer treatment and recovery, relationships with family and friends may have centered on your illness. Learning to refocus those relationships on other matters and a future together can take a new way of thinking. Reclaiming your place in your circle of friends may be difficult at first. Tell others how you feel and openly address their fears and questions.

Many of the old stigmas associated with cancer still exist. For example, you may have to remind co-workers that cancer isn't contagious and that cancer survivors can be just as productive as people without cancer.

There are also financial realities, such as insurance. If you experience difficulties switching or obtaining insurance, find out if your state provides health insurance for people who are difficult to insure. Look into group insurance options through professional, fraternal or political organizations.

Life after cancer can sometimes mean discarding old fears and uncertainties and facing new challenges. But as you adapt to these changes, you'll undoubtedly experience a sense of recovery and control.

Not all families are open and sharing. You or a family member may find it difficult to discuss feelings openly. Sometimes, it's easier to talk to someone outside your circle of friends, such as a counselor or cancer survivor.

Reach out to family and friends. You may think it should be the other way around. For some of your closest friends, it will be — they'll come to you. But recall people in your past who were ill and how hard it was to think of what to say or do to help them.

Find ways to put family and friends at ease. Inquire about the projects that a busy acquaintance has going. Invite someone who's not a great talker to help you with a chore. Be a willing listener for friends who have plenty of their own problems.

Accept help from others. It's difficult to fight cancer alone. Many times your family and friends are looking for clues that show them how to support you. If they say, "Let me know how I can help," go ahead and tell them — even if it's simply being on call for emotional support. Most people are grateful to have a chance to show you, in practical ways, that they care. All they need is an invitation.

Finding support

In the days and weeks after completing cancer treatment, you may feel as if you're suddenly alone in the world. Friends and family can help fill the void, but sometimes only fellow cancer survivors — people who've been there — can give you specifically what you need.

Cancer support groups bring together people who've had cancer. Participants talk about their own experiences and feelings, they listen to the concerns of others, and they discuss the challenges of life after cancer.

Is a support group right for you?

If you answer yes to most of the following questions, joining a cancer support group may be a positive step for you:

- Are you comfortable sharing feelings with others in a similar situation?
- Are you interested in hearing how others feel about their experiences?
- Could you benefit from the advice of other cancer survivors?
- Do you enjoy being part of a group?
- Do you have helpful information or hints to share with others?
- Would reaching out to help others with cancer give you satisfaction?
- Would you feel comfortable around others who may have different ways of dealing with their cancer?
- Are you interested in learning more about cancer issues?

Adapted from "Facing Forward: A Guide for Cancer Survivors," National Cancer Institute, National Institutes of Health, 2002

Not everyone needs a support group. Having family and friends may be all the support you need. But some may find it helpful to interact with people outside their immediate circles.

In general, support groups fall into two main categories — those led by health care professionals, such as a psychologist or nurse, and those led by group members themselves. Some are structured and educational. Others emphasize emotional support and shared experience. Some focus on a specific kind of cancer, while others involve a broader range of interests, including people with all types of cancer.

No matter how the support group is set up, the goal should be the same — how attending the meetings helps you cope and live better with cancer.

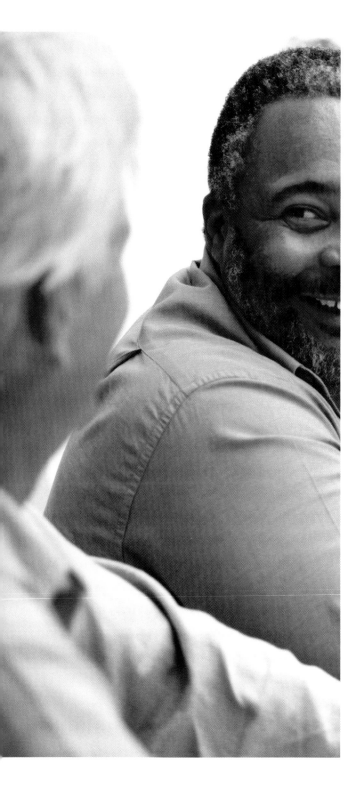

Benefits

The key to success with support groups is finding one that matches your needs and personality. The benefits you may receive include:

Sense of belonging. A special camaraderie often forms among group members. When you feel accepted in the group, you may also become more accepting of yourself.

Understanding. Support group members have firsthand knowledge of what you're experiencing without you having to explain it to them. You may express feelings without fear that you'll be misunderstood.

Exchange of advice. When group members talk, you know they speak from experience. They can describe coping techniques that have worked for them and those that haven't helped.

As a cautionary note, support groups may also include people offering opinions that are not well-founded, and are potentially harmful. It's always best to consider any advice in relation to information that you've received from other reliable sources. And consult your doctor before taking any actions.

The Internet offers online support groups but, in similar fashion, be careful about the reliability of the information you find — there's bound to be bad advice mixed in with what's good.

The disadvantage of online support groups is that you don't always know much about who is online with you. Avoid groups that promise a cure or claim to be a substitute for medical treatment. Look for groups affiliated with reputable organizations, or hosted by medical experts.

Friendship. Group members can bring joy into your life as well as practical support — a listening ear when you need to talk, a chauffeur when you could use a relaxing drive, and a companion to exercise with.

To gain the most benefit from a group setting, you need to find the meetings enjoyable. If you find them awkward or uncomfortable, trust your instincts and stop attending the meetings.

In addition, not all support groups are beneficial and positive. Some groups that aren't carefully monitored become a place to vent and share only negative feelings, which leaves you depressed and adds to your frustration.

Finding a support group

What support group you choose may depend largely on what's available in your local community. To find a group:

- Ask your doctor or other health care professional for assistance.
- Check your telephone directory or newspaper for a listing of support resources.
- Contact community centers, libraries or religious organizations.
- Ask others you know who have or had cancer.
- Contact a national cancer organization such as the American Cancer Society at 800-227-2345, or Cancer Care at 800-813-4673.

Most support groups are free, collect voluntary donations or charge only modest dues to cover expenses.

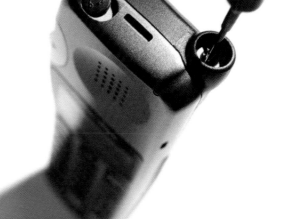

Answers to your questions

What if, months after treatment, a PSA test produces an elevated reading? Does this mean the cancer is back?

If you still have your prostate gland, an elevated PSA level can be normal or it may indicate that the cancer is progressing. Elevated PSA levels after removal of the prostate usually indicate that cancer is present.

How long will it take after surgery before I can exercise and take part in sporting activities again?

Fatigue can linger for three to six months after surgery. Your ability to participate also depends on the activity and your physical condition before surgery. Somewhere between six weeks and two months after surgery you may be able to jog, golf, swim or play tennis at a leisurely pace. It may be many months, however, before you can ride a bicycle or a horse. A bicycle seat or a saddle places pressure on the lower pelvis, the location of the surgery.

What's a living will?

A living will is also referred to as an advance directive. It's a legal document that states your wishes about your medical care in case of a terminal illness. For example, it states whether you want to be placed on a breathing device (ventilator) or have a feeding tube. If you choose to prepare a living will, it's important that people in charge of your care, such as your doctor and a family member, receive copies.

Does the fear that the cancer will return ever go away?

Some people who have had successful treatment are able to get past this fear. Others aren't. But in most cases, the fear wanes as the months and years pass. No one expects you to forget you've had cancer. But your fears will become fewer and farther between as you fill your mind and time with other thoughts and activities.

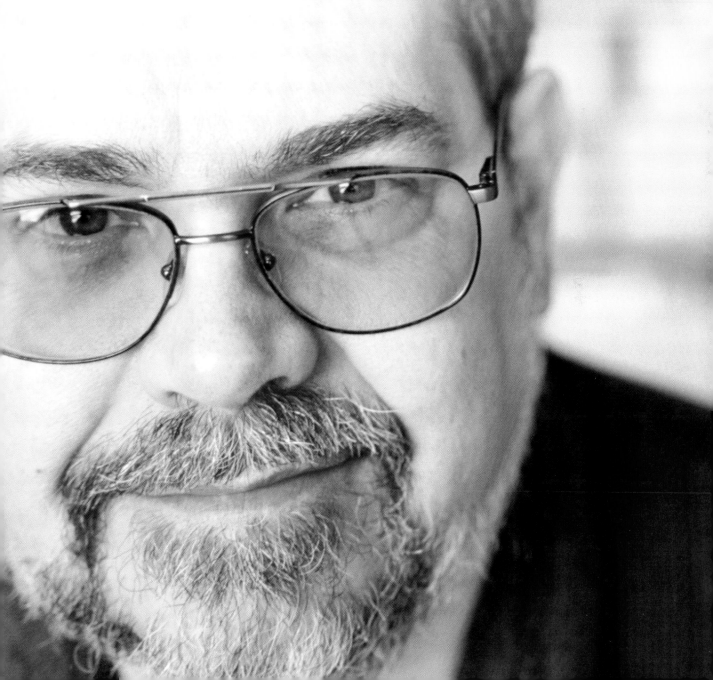

Part 4

Prostate health

Chapter 11

Can you prevent prostate disease?

The changes taking place in your prostate as you age are a result of many factors, including genetics, environment and physical health. Although prostate disorders are a common problem for men, that doesn't mean they're inevitable. The combination of factors that may cause prostate problems varies from person to person, similar to the variety of ways that prostate symptoms may impact quality of life.

True, there's no formula guaranteeing that you won't get prostate disease. But there are definite actions you can take to reduce your risk, or possibly slow progression of the disease.

Three important steps that can help you maintain your prostate health also turn out to be excellent steps for maintaining general health. These are simple, not uncommon measures, and hopefully, you've been practicing them for many years:
- Eat well
- Keep physically active
- See your doctor regularly

How much benefit you'll receive by taking these steps is unknown. There's no way to know if they'll actually prevent prostate inflammation, enlargement or cancer, but they will make your body stronger and healthier.

Potential cancer-fighting foods

Researchers are examining certain foods and beverages to see if they might help reduce your risk of prostate disease, especially cancer. Although studies to this point have been inconclusive, some results look promising. These foods, regardless, can be part of a healthy diet, and you should have few concerns about including them in meals.

Antioxidant-rich foods

Antioxidants are substances that protect your body's cells from the effects of free radicals — unstable molecules that turn toxic when they're produced in over-abundance. Free radical damage to the prostate may cause cancer. Antioxidants help stabilize the molecules, reducing the damage they could cause.

Recent studies have been inconclusive so far and have not established a direct link between the antioxidant properties of certain foods and the prevention of disease. Nevertheless, increasing your intake of foods rich in antioxidants appears to improve your nutrition and enhance your overall health.

Antioxidants are found in many vegetables and fruits, especially those with intense color — red, purple, blue, orange and yellow. Other sources of antioxidants are nuts, grains and some meats, poultry and fish.

Beta carotene is an antioxidant found in foods that are orange in color, including carrots, squash, cantaloupe, apricots and mangos. Lutein (LOO-te-in) is found in dark green leafy vegetables, such as spinach and kale.

Tomatoes and tomato products contain lycopene (LY-ko-pene), an antioxidant that gives the fruit its red color. Studies have shown that there's more antioxidants in cooked tomato products — soups as well as sauces used in spaghetti and pizza — than in raw products such as fresh tomatoes or tomato juice. On the other hand, broccoli provides more antioxidants in its raw form than in its cooked form.

It's important not to overdo your intake to avoid consuming an excessive amount of antioxidants. Consumption beyond your body's ability to use them could lead to increased production of free radicals. In addition, it's probably best to get your antioxidants from food rather than from supplements.

Vitamins and minerals

Research on the role of vitamins and minerals in preventing prostate cancer is inconclusive — while some studies suggest they may reduce risk, others indicate no such benefit. Several studies have focused on whether vitamins C, D, E and the mineral selenium help prevent prostate disease.

A major study funded in part by the National Cancer Institute was halted recently when it was determined that vitamin E and selenium, taken alone or together, showed no evidence of preventing prostate cancer. Furthermore, researchers discovered a slight increase in developing prostate cancer among participants taking only vitamin E and a slight increase in developing diabetes among participants taking only selenium.

Researchers also are investigating the effect of the mineral zinc on prostate health. Zinc is most abundant in meat, seafood, poultry and whole grains. The prostate gland contains more zinc than does any other organ, and research suggests that too little zinc may contribute to prostate disease.

Most doctors don't recommend taking individual supplements for the sole purpose of reducing your risk of prostate disease. Not enough is known about their role in preventing disease, or at what dosage they should be taken — high doses of some vitamins and minerals may be toxic. If you believe your diet isn't giving you all the nutrients you need, there's little harm in taking a daily multivitamin. But many doctors will encourage you to get vitamins and minerals through whole foods, and to not exceed the recommended dietary allowances.

Sources of soy

Soy isn't a common ingredient in foods, but you can find items containing soy in well-stocked grocery and health food stores:

Dried soybeans. Soak the beans overnight and then cook to soften. You may also find precooked products. Add the beans to your favorite recipes, including soups, chilis, stir-fries or salads.

Tofu. Its neutral taste and spongy texture make it ideal for absorbing other flavors. Substitute it in place of meat for a main course.

Tempeh and miso. Tempeh is available in a thin cake, and miso is a paste. Both can be used in soups and salads or as a meat substitute.

Textured soy protein (TSP). Available in the frozen-food section, TSP is found in soy burgers and can be used in casseroles or foods such as tacos.

Soy milk. Use it in recipes or on cereal.

Soy flour. Can be substituted for a portion of all-purpose flour in many baked goods. You also can substitute 1 tablespoon of soy flour and 1 to 2 tablespoons of water for each egg in baking recipes.

Soy

The soybean is a legume native to northern China and now commonly grown in the United States. Fermentation techniques allow soy to be prepared in a variety of forms, including tempeh, miso, tofu and tamari (soy) sauce.

Active compounds in soy (isoflavones) appear to help keep the sex hormones testosterone and estrogen in check. Because prostate cancer cells feed off testosterone, researchers theorize that reducing the hormone's effect may lower your risk of cancer.

In Asia, where soy is a food staple, certain types of cancers, including prostate and breast cancers, are less common. However, it's uncertain whether this benefit is due to soy or to some other aspect of Asian lifestyle — for example, the Asian diet is much lower in fat than is the typical American diet.

There's some evidence that isoflavones in soy may lower your risk of benign prostatic hyperplasia (BPH). Soy also provides fiber, vitamins and minerals, and is a great source of dietary protein minus all the fat and cholesterol found in meat. But claims that soy can reduce cholesterol levels are unconfirmed.

Green tea

Green tea contains polyphenols — compounds with strong antioxidant qualities. One such polyphenol is epigallocatechin gallate (EGCG), which may play a role in cancer prevention by suppressing the activity of enzymes necessary for cancer growth.

However, it's unclear from research studies whether other lifestyle factors may have played significant, if not greater, roles in achieving these results. Furthermore, large daily consumption was required in order for the tea to register any benefits.

While the preventive possibilities of green tea remain promising, it doesn't appear to help treat cancer. A Mayo Clinic study found no evidence that green tea helped men with advanced prostate cancer that had become resistant to hormone therapy. In addition, most participants experienced disruptive side effects from consuming high daily amounts of green tea.

Although all of the benefits of green tea still haven't been thoroughly studied, the beverage does appear to have some medicinal qualities and doesn't pose serious complications.

Dairy products and prostate cancer

According to the American Institute for Cancer Research (AICR), debate continues regarding a link between milk consumption and prostate cancer. Some studies indicate that a high-calcium intake — primarily from dairy products — may slightly increase the cancer risk. Researchers theorize that the extra calcium suppresses a hormone believed to protect against cancer.

The AICR notes that the calcium intake in these studies was well above the recommended daily intake. Because of the important nutrients in dairy products, the AICR suggests that men have a balanced diet including two servings of low-fat or fat-free dairy products daily to maintain calcium at safer levels. More research is needed to determine whether calcium or fat or some other component in dairy products may be responsible for the increased risk.

Cruciferous vegetables

Cruciferous vegetables include bok choy, broccoli, Brussels sprouts, cabbage, cauliflower, collards, rutabagas and turnips. Although studies haven't established a link between dietary intake and cancer prevention, they do suggest that regularly eating cruciferous vegetables may provide some benefits during the earliest stages of tumor growth, before the cancer is detectable.

Garlic

In regions of the world where people eat a lot of garlic, there tends to be less prostate cancer. However, study results have been inconclusive, and some studies have used multi-ingredient products, making it difficult to know if garlic alone has produced the modest benefit. Regardless, you should have no worries about including garlic in your diet to enhance the flavor of cooking.

Controlling calories and fat

Several studies have suggested that a link may exist between having a high-calorie, high-fat diet and developing prostate cancer.

One study from the Fred Hutchinson Cancer Research Center, Seattle, suggests that a high-calorie intake may lead to a higher risk of localized prostate cancer (stays within the prostate) and nonlocalized prostate cancer (spreads outside the prostate). They also found a link between high-fat diets and nonlocalized prostate cancer.

However, key questions from this research remain unanswered. It's uncertain whether the relationship between high-fat intake and cancer is due to the amount of fat or to a specific type of fat. Complicating this analysis is the fact that it's often difficult to distinguish between the separate effects that fat and calories may have on cancer.

Until these questions are addressed, the basic message is, the less fat and the fewer calories you consume, the better your diet.

The food groups

The food groups of the Mayo Clinic Healthy Weight Pyramid include vegetables, fruits, carbohydrates, protein and dairy, fats, and sweets. The pyramid promotes a plant-based diet — the vegetable and fruit groups share the base of the pyramid, with carbohydrates, including foods made with whole grains, located above them.

Eating more plant-based foods is the best way to reduce fat and calories in your diet — many plant foods are virtually fat-free. Plant foods also are loaded with vitamins, minerals, fiber, antioxidants and cancer-protective compounds called phytochemicals.

Here are descriptions of each food group and recommended daily servings from the Healthy Weight Pyramid:

Vegetables and fruits: At least 7 to 10 servings. Eating more vegetables and fruits may be one of the best things you can do to improve your health. Fresh vegetables and fruits have a low energy density, meaning there's relatively few calories in a large volume of food. You can eat almost unlimited amounts from these two food groups without worrying about weight.

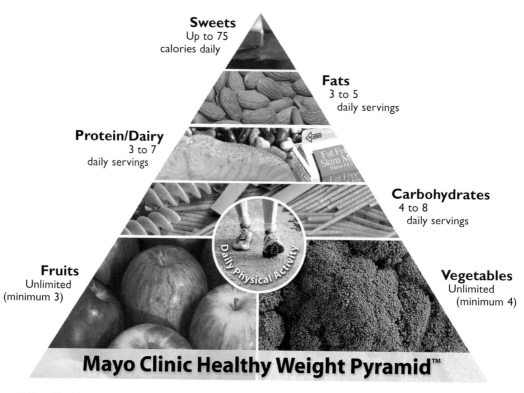

Sweets
Up to 75
calories daily

Fats
3 to 5
daily servings

Protein/Dairy
3 to 7
daily servings

Carbohydrates
4 to 8
daily servings

Fruits
Unlimited
(minimum 3)

Daily Physical Activity

Vegetables
Unlimited
(minimum 4)

Mayo Clinic Healthy Weight Pyramid™

© Mayo Foundation for Medical Education and Research.
See your doctor before you begin any healthy weight plan.

The Mayo Clinic Healthy Weight Pyramid is your guide for achieving and maintaining a healthy diet. Its triangular shape shows you where to focus your attention when selecting healthy foods. You want to eat more from the food groups at the base of the pyramid and less from those at the top.

The number of servings you should consume from each food group is based on your daily calorie goals. When a range of servings is shown with a particular food group, the lower number of servings is based on 1,200 daily calories and the higher number is based on 2,000 daily calories. Note that servings of fruits and vegetables are unlimited because these foods are so low in calories and fat.

The circle at the center of the pyramid stresses the importance of daily physical activity in helping you maintain a healthy diet and healthy weight.

In addition to being virtually fat-free and low in calories, vegetables and fruits provide fiber, phytochemicals and a variety of nutrients, including potassium and magnesium, that are necessary for good health.

Substituting fruits and vegetables for foods that have more fat and calories is a relatively easy way to improve your diet without cutting back on the amount you eat. The key is not to smother your food with dips or sauces that contain a lot of fat.

Fresh fruit is best, but frozen fruits with no added sugar or fruits canned in their own juice or water also are excellent. Use fruit juice and dried fruits sparingly because they're concentrated sources of calories. That is, they have a higher energy density.

Carbohydrates: 4 to 8 servings. This group includes a wide range of foods that are a major energy source for your body. Most carbohydrates are plant based. These include grain products such as breads, cereals, rice and pasta. Other food groups providing carbohydrates include starchy vegetables such as potatoes, corn and squash. Dairy products are the only animal-based foods that supply carbohydrates.

When choosing grain products, look for the word *whole* — as in whole wheat — on the packaging. Whole grains contain the bran and the germ, which are sources of fiber, vitamins and minerals, such as magnesium. When grains are refined, some of the nutrients and the fiber have been eliminated. As a rule, the less refined a carbohydrate is, the better it is for you.

Carbohydrates are generally low in fat and calories, but products may vary in energy density. For example, select plain yeast breads rather than dessert breads, sweet rolls or other baked goods, which may be loaded with sugary ingredients. Be selective about what you add to these foods. Use vegetable or fresh tomato-based sauces on pasta and avoid cream and cheese sauces.

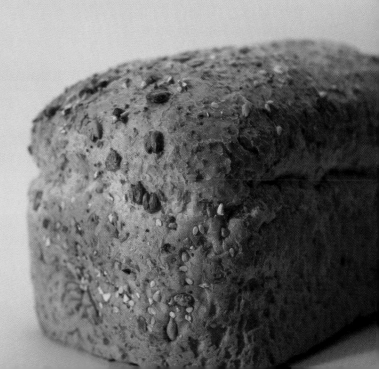

Protein and dairy: 3 to 7 servings. Proteins are in every living cell in your body, performing many vital roles in cell function. For good health, you should eat some protein every day. Americans tend to have a protein-heavy diet, and most easily meet or exceed their daily requirement.

This food group has both plant and animal sources. Plant-based foods rich in protein — and relatively low in fat — include beans, peas and lentils. Animal-based foods rich in protein include fish and seafood, poultry, meat, eggs and dairy products such as milk, cheese and yogurt. Choose lean meat, poultry without skin, fish, and low-fat or fat-free dairy products to reduce your fat and calorie intake.

Fats: 3 to 5 servings. Many people are surprised to hear that fats are important for good health. Believe it or not, you always need to include some fat in your diet.

But not all fats are equal. The healthier fats are monounsaturated, including olive oil, canola oil, nuts and nut products, and avocados. Polyunsaturated fats include safflower, corn, sunflower and soy oils, and can be found in varieties of cold-water fish such as salmon.

Saturated fats and trans fats are less healthy. Saturated fats are found in red meats, whole-fat dairy products, butter, lard, coconut oil and other tropical oils. Trans fats are used in commercially produced products such as cookies, pastries, crackers and deep-fried foods.

All fats contain approximately 45 calories a serving and are a high-energy-density food. For that reason, all fats, including the healthier ones, should be consumed sparingly. An obvious way to cut fat in your diet is to reduce the amount of butter, margarine and vegetable oil that you add during cooking.

Sweets and alcohol: Sparingly. Cakes, cookies, pastries and other desserts are high sources of calories — mostly from sugar and fat — but offer little in terms of nutrition. You don't have to give up these foods entirely, but be smart about your selections and portion sizes. Better dessert choices include a small square of dark chocolate, fig bar cookie or low-fat frozen yogurt.

Alcohol also provides calories but no nutrients. According to the American Cancer Society, heavy alcohol consumption may cause certain types of cancer — although prostate cancer does not appear to be one of these types. However, the regular consumption of alcohol often replaces healthier dietary options that you could include in your regular meals. If you do drink alcohol, it's best to do so in moderation — no more than two drinks a day for an adult male.

Daily calorie goals

Theoretically, if what you eat contains the same number of calories as what you burn each day, you'll maintain your weight because you're eating exactly as many calories as your body requires. For most people, this ranges between 1,600 and 2,400 daily calories. But in practice, people often eat more calories than they realize (and exercise less than they think). If you're uncertain of your daily calorie goal, your doctor can help you.

The recommended servings for food groups from the Mayo Clinic Healthy Weight Pyramid can guide your decision making and help you stay within your daily calorie goals. But these recommendations may need to be adapted to your individual needs. For example, over time your calorie goals may change based on age, health risks and activity level. You can adjust the serving totals accordingly.

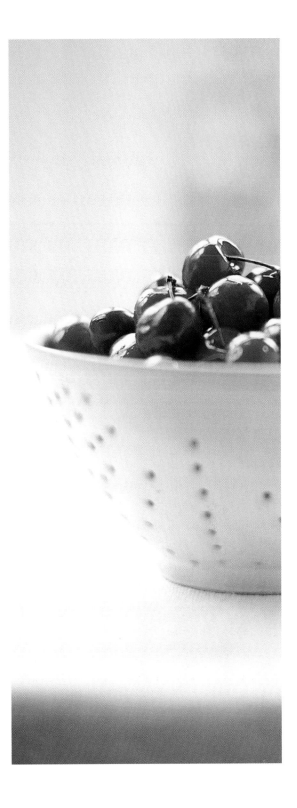

Being active

It's well known that regular exercise can promote cardiovascular health, giving you more energy and helping prevent heart attacks and conditions such as high blood pressure and high cholesterol. When it comes to preventing cancer, the data aren't as clear-cut. However, studies indicate that regular exercise may help reduce cancer risk, including prostate cancer.

Regular exercise has been shown to strengthen your immune system, improve circulation and speed digestion — all of which may play a role in cancer prevention. Exercise also helps prevent obesity, another potential risk factor for some cancers.

As well, men who are physically active usually develop less severe symptoms of benign prostatic hyperplasia (BPH) than do men who get little exercise. Regular exercise also may help reduce your risk of BPH.

However, you may want to increase your activity gradually. If you're recovering from surgery or other medical treatment, talk with your doctor before beginning a physical activity program.

Are you fit?

Federal guidelines generally recommend that you get between 30 and 60 minutes of moderate physical activity every day. But, according to a Surgeon General report, more than 60 percent of American adults aren't active on a regular basis and, worse yet, 25 percent aren't active at all.

Simply put, most Americans are not physically fit. Being fit allows you to function in daily life and maintain good health, reducing your risk of many medical conditions. To know if you're fit, consider these indicators:

- You have enough energy to enjoy the activities you want to do.
- You have no problem carrying out the daily tasks of life.
- You can hold a conversation while doing light to moderate exercise.
- You can walk a mile without feeling winded or fatigued.
- You easily climb three flights of stairs.

You're probably not as fit as you should be if you're feeling tired most of the time, not being able to keep up with others your age, and becoming short of breath or fatigued when you walk a short distance.

Before you get started

It's a good idea to talk with your doctor before starting a physical activity program. If you have another health problem or you're at risk of heart disease, you may need to take special precautions while you exercise. It's important to see your doctor if you:

- Have blood pressure of 140/90 millimeters of mercury or higher
- Have diabetes or heart, lung or kidney disease
- Are 40 years or older and haven't had a recent physical examination
- Have a family history of heart-related problems before age 55
- Are unsure of your health status
- Have experienced chest discomfort, shortness of breath or dizziness during exercise or strenuous activity

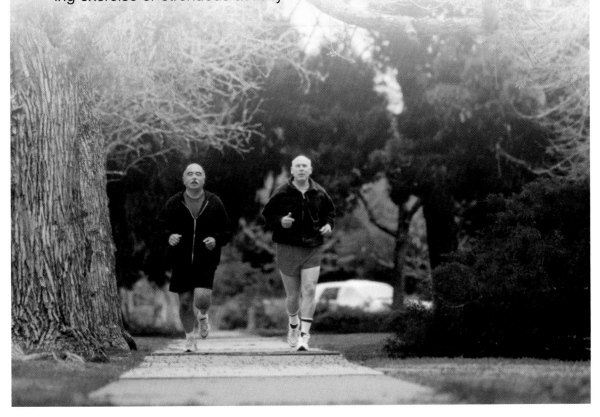

How hard are you exercising?

How do you know if the activity you're doing is moderate exercise? The Borg ratings of perceived exertion scale is one way to estimate exercise intensity. *Perceived exertion* refers to the total amount of effort and stress you feel during an activity, including heart rate, breathing rate, perspiration and muscle fatigue.

The scale ranges from 6 (your body at rest) to 20 (maximal effort). You gauge the perceived effort while you exercise — moderate activity ranges from 11 to 14. Your perception of exercise intensity is more important than your absolute level of exertion. For example, brisk walking benefits a person who's in shape as well as a person who's out of shape, but they'll be walking at a different pace for what each perceives as moderate exercise.

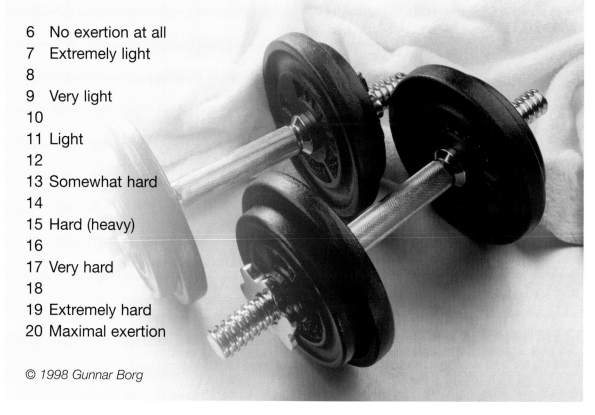

6   No exertion at all
7   Extremely light
8
9   Very light
10
11 Light
12
13 Somewhat hard
14
15 Hard (heavy)
16
17 Very hard
18
19 Extremely hard
20 Maximal exertion

© 1998 Gunnar Borg

How to shape up

You can improve your fitness, regardless of your age and weight or the condition of your health. But exercising, if you haven't been active in the recent past, can be a big change. Many people start an exercise program but don't stick with it — often because they try to do too much too soon. This all-or-nothing mentality is a recipe for discouragement, not to mention possible injury.

It's better to start a program gradually, at a pace that you're comfortable with. Even the most inactive people can benefit from adding just a few minutes more of physical activity each day.

There are different types of exercise, and each type affects your body in a different way. Some exercises are designed to strengthen your heart while others build endurance. Some help keep you flexible while others build bone and muscle mass.

Typically, an exercise program consists of the three major types of exercise: aerobic, flexibility and strength training. Combining this program with a healthy diet can provide you with many health benefits — possibly helping to prevent prostate disease or reduce its symptoms.

Aerobic exercises. Aerobic activities improve your cardiovascular fitness — the health of your heart, lungs and circulatory system. This increases your ability to use oxygen, referred to as aerobic capacity. A higher aerobic capacity gives you more endurance and allows you to work at a more intense level for a longer time. Aerobic exercise burns a lot of calories and is, therefore, excellent for meeting weight goals.

Try to do at least 30 minutes of aerobic exercise on most, if not all, days of the week. But your activity doesn't have to be condensed into one chunk of time — the cumulative effect of physical activity is what matters. If you can't exercise for 30 minutes at a time, aim for three 10-minute sessions.

Brisk walking is the most common aerobic exercise because it's easy, convenient and inexpensive. All you need is a good pair of walking shoes. Walk at an even, comfortable pace that you can maintain. If you're getting short of breath, slow down.

Once you're able to walk a few miles without much strain, you can vary the intensity by walking hills, lengthening your stride, swinging your arms more or increasing your speed.

If brisk walking doesn't appeal to you, you can choose other kinds of aerobic activity. Choose a type of exercise that appeals to you — you're more likely to stick with a program that's fun. Aerobic exercise also includes:

- Bicycling
- Swimming
- Jogging
- Tennis and other racket sports
- Golfing (when walking, not riding)
- Dancing
- Basketball
- Volleyball
- Water aerobics
- Cross-country skiing

Flexibility exercises. Stretching before and after aerobic activity increases the range in which you can bend and stretch your joints, muscles and ligaments. Flexibility exercises also help prevent joint pain and injury.

The stretches should be gentle and slow. Stretch only until you feel slight tension in your muscles. If a stretch hurts, you've gone too far — ease up. Relax and breathe freely. Don't hold your breath while stretching.

If you have time to stretch only once, stretch after your workout because your muscles will be warmed up.

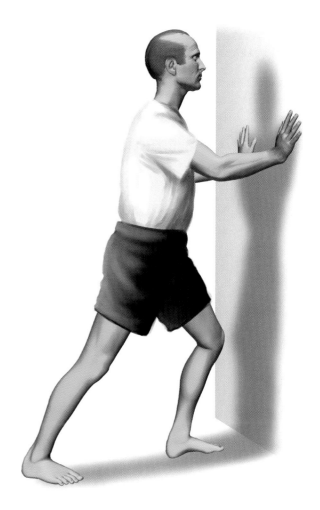

Calf stretch

Stand at arm's length from the wall. Lean your upper body into the wall. Place one leg forward with knee bent. Keep your other leg back with your knee straight and your heel down. Keeping your back straight, move your hips toward the wall until you feel a stretch. Hold for 30 seconds. Relax. Repeat with the other leg.

Upper-thigh stretch

Lie on your back on a table or bed, with one leg and hip as near the edge as possible. Let your lower leg hang relaxed over the edge. Grasp the knee of your other leg, and pull your thigh and knee firmly toward your chest until your lower back flattens against the table or bed. Hold for 30 seconds. Relax. Repeat with the other leg.

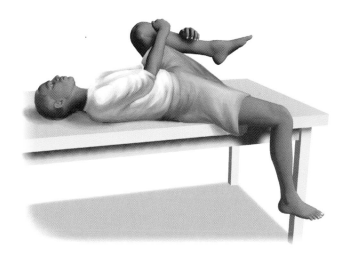

Chest stretch

Clasp your hands behind your head. Pull your elbows firmly back while inhaling deeply. Hold for 30 seconds. Relax.

Low back stretch

Lie flat on a firm surface. With your knees bent, lift one leg at a time toward your body. Grasp your knees and pull toward your shoulders. Stop when you feel a stretch in your lower back. Hold. Return legs, one at a time, to starting position. Repeat. Avoid this exercise if you have osteoporosis or an artificial hip implant.

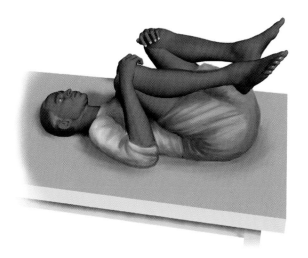

Strength training. When it comes to overall fitness, investing in a set of weights or resistance bands may pay dividends as great as those gained with a pair of walking shoes. Strength training reduces body fat and increases lean muscle mass — allowing you to burn calories more efficiently. These exercises also help improve posture and balance, and promote healthy bones. Some strengthening exercises are shown on these pages.

Strength training involves working your muscles against some form of resistance. When your muscles push or pull against a force such as gravity, a free weight or your own body weight, they grow stronger.

Sessions lasting 20 to 30 minutes and two to three times a week are sufficient for most people. Start with five repetitions of each exercise and try to build up to 12 repetitions.

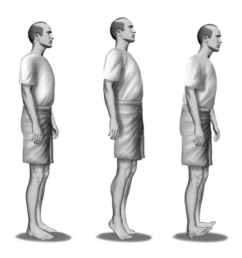

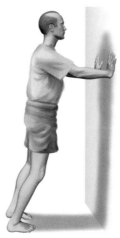

Toe and heel raise

Standing, rise up so that your weight is on your toes. Then rock back and shift your weight to your heels, lifting your toes off the ground. This strengthens your calf and lower leg muscles to improve your balance.

Wall push-ups

Place your palms on the wall with your elbows slightly bent. Slowly bend your elbows and lean toward the wall, supporting your body weight with your arms. Straighten your arms and return to your starting position.

Stretch your muscles before and after each workout. Complete all movements slowly and with complete control, and maintain normal breathing patterns. If you're unable to maintain good form and breathing, decrease the resistance (weight) or the repetitions. If the exercise causes pain, stop.

Because strength training contributes to better balance, coordination and agility, it may help prevent falls.

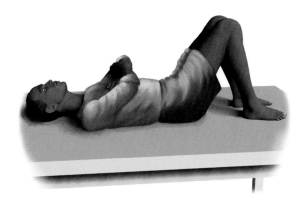

Abdominal exercise No. 1

Lie on a firm surface with your knees bent. Flatten the small of your back against the surface and concentrate on tightening your abdominal muscles. Relax and repeat.

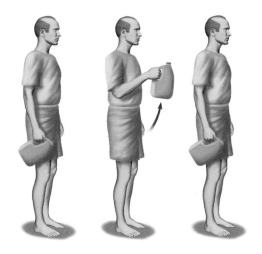

Arm curl

Hold a partially filled half-gallon milk jug. Flex your elbow until your hand reaches shoulder height. Hold, then lower your arm slowly. Remember to keep your wrist rigid while lifting — don't bend or curl your wrist.

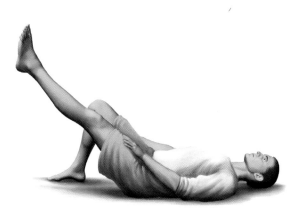

Abdominal exercise No. 2

Lie on your back with your right knee bent and your left knee straight. Hold your abdominal muscles tight, and slowly raise and lower your left leg. Relax and repeat. Reverse legs. Avoid doing this abdominal exercise if you have osteoporosis.

Staying active

About half the people who start an exercise program will drop out within six months. Some stop when they get bored or think the results come too slowly. Others overdo exercise and quickly become discouraged by the muscle pain and stiffness they feel after a workout.

The following tips may help you stay motivated and involved:

Be patient. It's better to progress slowly than to push too hard and be forced to abandon your program because of pain or injury. Improvements may not develop overnight, but you'll notice a difference within about a month.

It generally takes about three months for an exercise program to become routine. If you can stay with your program for that long, you're more likely to continue it and enjoy the activity.

Make it fun. Boredom is a major reason why people stop exercising. You're more likely to stay with your program if you choose activities you enjoy. Work out with a friend or join a fitness class. Listen to music, watch television or read while you work out.

Add variety. Alternating between different activities reduces your chance of injury from overusing a muscle or joint. It also keeps things more interesting. For example, you might alternate walking with bicycling, swimming or a low-impact aerobics class. On days when the weather is pleasant, do your flexibility exercises outside.

Suit your personality and lifestyle. If you prefer solitude, you may enjoy walking or bicycling. If group activities appeal to you, consider enrolling in a dance class or bowling league. Plan exercise for a time of day that suits you best, and make it convenient. Even if you prefer exercising outdoors, you can still plan indoor activities in case of bad weather.

Avoid all-or-nothing thinking. If you can't do your usual workout, do what you can. On days when time is tight or your motivation is waning, do less, but do *something*.

Get support. Encouragement from family and friends can be motivating. Studies show that social support helps people stay with their programs. Exercising with a partner helps you get out the door on those days when you're not inspired.

Track your progress. An exercise diary shows you what you've accomplished and helps you set goals for the future. Record what you do each time you exercise, how long you do it, and how you feel during and after exercising. Seeing your progress in writing can be a powerful motivator.

Reward yourself. Work on developing an internal sense of reward based on feelings of accomplishment, self-esteem and self-control. After each activity session, take a few minutes to sit down and relax. Savor the good feelings that exercise gives you and reflect on what goals you've just accomplished.

Be flexible with your schedule. If you're tired, feel a cold coming on or have a hectic day, don't force yourself to work out. Take the day off, and continue your program as soon as you're feeling better.

Expect lapses. There will be days when you move less than you had intended — or you skip the workout entirely. That's what's called a lapse, and it's inevitable that you'll occasionally lapse. Don't use a lapse as an excuse to give up. A brief period of time when you can't exercise isn't a disaster. Just get going as soon as you can.

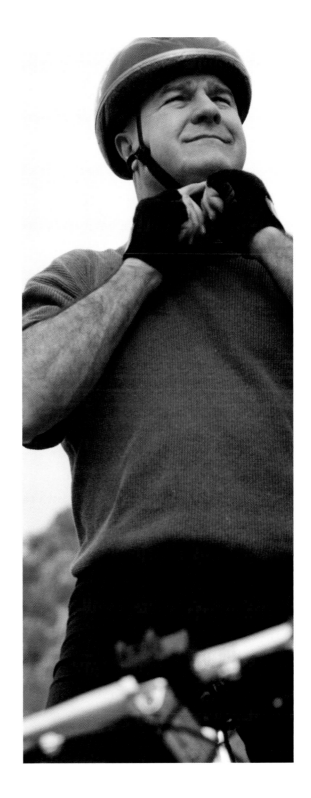

Reducing the risks of exercise

Most risks of exercise stem from doing too much, too vigorously, with too little previous conditioning. To reduce risks:

Start out slowly. Don't overdo it. Gradually increase your time and pace. To build up to 30 minutes, start with 10 minutes, and increase your time in five-minute increments. If you have trouble talking to a companion during your workout, you're probably pushing too hard.

Exercise regularly and moderately. Never exercise to the point of nausea, dizziness, severe shortness of breath, heart palpitations, or tightness or pain in your chest. If you experience any of these symptoms, stop exercising and get immediate medical care.

Always warm up and cool down. This reduces stress on your heart and muscles.

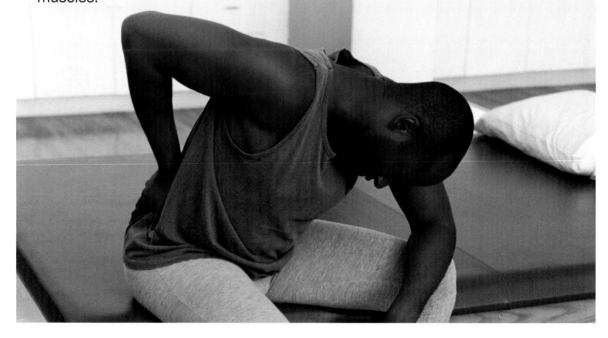

Seeing your doctor regularly

Annual prostate exams can't reduce your risk of cancer, BPH or prostatitis, as perhaps a healthy diet or regular physical exercise may be able to do. But these regular checkups are still crucial to staying healthy.

If prostate disease does develop, a digital rectal exam or prostate-specific antigen (PSA) test often can catch the problem in its earliest stages — when many conditions are easier to treat and cure. If you don't regularly see a doctor, schedule an appointment to have a general physical examination, including a prostate exam, and make it a yearly habit.

If you notice prostate-related signs and symptoms — for example, if you experience increased urination, difficulty urinating, pain while urinating, lower pelvic and back pain, or blood in your urine or semen — schedule a visit with your doctor. Have the problem attended to as soon as possible, even if you believe that it's not a big deal. You don't want to risk the possibility that you could be wrong.

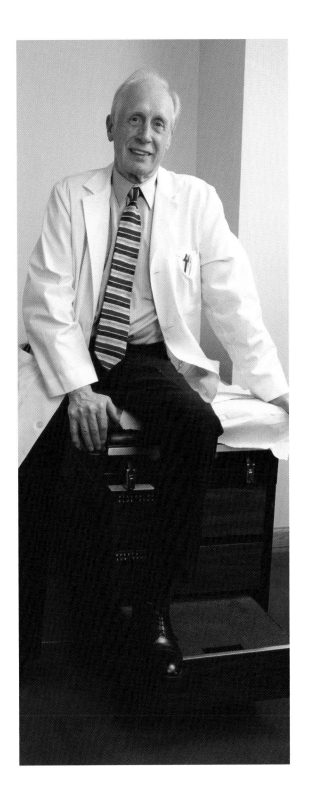

Answers to your questions

Does alcohol play a role in the risk of prostate disease?

There's no evidence that a moderate amount of alcohol causes prostate disease. A moderate amount of alcohol for men is two drinks a day — one drink a day if you're 65 or older. However, if you regularly drink more than a moderate amount of alcohol, this may interfere with your diet. People who drink excessive amounts of alcohol often substitute alcohol for food and may not get adequate amounts of nutrients. A poor diet can weaken your immune system and reduce your body's natural defenses against disease.

Is soy sauce a good source of soy?

No. Soy sauce doesn't contain beneficial amounts of cancer-fighting chemicals, and it's very high in sodium. If you're sensitive to sodium, regular use of soy sauce can increase your blood pressure.

Is it true that stress can cause prostate problems?

It hasn't been proved that stress increases your risk of prostate disease, but there's some evidence that stress may play a role. Stress weakens your immune system, making it more difficult for your body to fight off disease, including cancer. Researchers also theorize that stress can produce tension in your lower pelvic muscles, affecting normal functioning of the prostate gland and, possibly, causing prostatitis.

Chapter 12

Complementary and alternative therapies

As Americans take a more active role in their health care, many are exploring options that are generally not considered part of conventional medical practice. These options, which include a broad range of healing philosophies, approaches and therapies such as dietary supplements, acupuncture, meditation and ayurveda, are referred to collectively as complementary and alternative medicine (CAM).

The National Center for Complementary and Alternative Medicine (NCCAM), a division of the National Institutes of Health, makes a distinction that "complementary" refers to treatments that

you might choose *in addition to* conventional medicine. For example, using tai chi in addition to prescription drugs to manage anxiety. In contrast, "alternative" refers to treatment that you might choose *in place of* conventional medicine. For example, seeing a homeopathic practitioner for your health care instead of a family physician.

There are legitimate concerns regarding many CAM products and practices that should be addressed before you consider using one of them. Some therapies haven't been studied adequately using accepted scientific methods. Often there's conflicting evidence as to

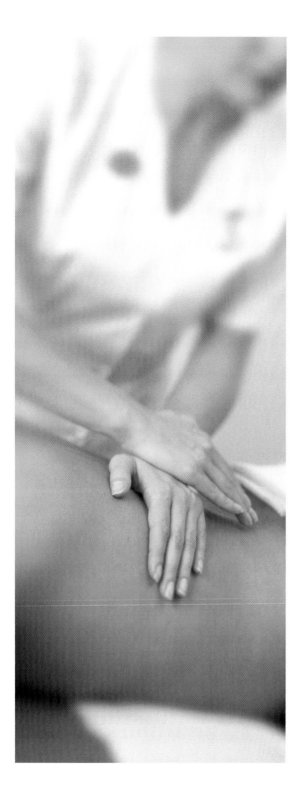

whether a treatment actually works or not — and, if so, how well and for how long. There's legitimate concerns about quality control, dosage, side effects and negative interactions with other medications you may be taking.

Even so, as young and old alike seek greater control of their own health care — either by choice or by circumstance — complementary and alternative therapies have become increasingly popular. And a growing body of evidence suggests that some CAM treatments may provide benefits and help you manage prostate health.

Integrative medicine is a fairly new term that describes a change taking place in many health care institutions — integrating CAM therapies with conventional medicine. The goal is to treat the whole person — mind, body and spirit — not just the disease. This is done by combining the best of today's high-tech medicine with the best of nontraditional practices that have high-quality evidence to support their use.

Here's a look at some of the more common complementary and alternative treatments that are promoted for the prevention or treatment of prostate disease, and for cancer in general.

Dietary supplements

As anyone who has walked through a health food store can attest, the profusion of dietary supplements is almost overwhelming. Literally thousands of products crowd the shelves, touting all sorts of claims.

Most dietary supplements are derived from plants or herbs, though minerals, vitamins and even some hormones are included in the category. Supplements — especially the herbal products — are popular because of the perception that they're natural and, therefore, "good for you."

Being natural doesn't always translate into being safe. Any product that's strong enough to provide a potential benefit to the body can also be strong enough to cause harm. Despite these concerns, certain supplements may be part of your overall wellness plan, provided you use them wisely.

Remember, supplements are just that — supplemental. They can't replace a nutritious diet, exercising every day and getting enough rest.

Herbal products that are marketed to relieve common prostate problems — such as frequent urination or weak urine flow — include:
- Pygeum (*Pygeum africanum*): also known as African plum tree
- African wild potato (*Hypoxis rooperi*): also known as South African star grass
- Pumpkin (*Cucurbita pepo*) seeds
- Rye grass (*Secale cereale*)
- The above-ground parts of stinging nettle (*Urtica dioica* and *Urtica urens*), also known as common nettle

If taken in small to moderate amounts, these products appear safe to use. However, they haven't been studied in large, long-term trials to verify their safety or to prove they actually work.

An exception may be the herb saw palmetto (*Serenoa repens*). Unlike other herbal supplements, it has been widely tested, and the results show more promise.

Saw palmetto

Saw palmetto products are made from the berries of this dwarf palm plant, which thrives in the warm climates of southeastern United States. Saw palmetto has become a popular treatment for reducing the symptoms of benign prostatic hyperplasia (BPH). In Europe, it's sold as a drug. In the United States, it's often available as a dietary supplement in health food stores.

Some researchers believe saw palmetto affects testosterone, the sex hormone believed to stimulate tissue growth in the prostate — although this interaction is still debated. Several studies have suggested that saw palmetto can help reduce abnormal growth in the prostate that obstructs the urethra, thereby increasing urine flow and improving overall quality of life.

However, a more recent trial found no significant benefits from taking the supplement. This isn't to say that the herb isn't effective, but it does suggest the need for more research to better understand its benefits.

Saw palmetto is generally safe when used as directed and side effects are rare, but you shouldn't use it if you have a bleeding problem.

Saw palmetto generally works slowly. Most men begin to see improvements within one to three months. If there's no benefits after three months, the product may not work for you.

Cancer fighters

Several dietary supplements claim to help cure or prevent cancer. There's no scientific evidence that these products can accomplish this, and some of the claims may even be dangerous. Two popular supplements that are sold as cancer-fighting agents are:

Chaparral. Also known as creosote bush or greasewood, chaparral (*Larrea tridentata*) comes from a desert shrub found in the southwestern United States and Mexico. American Indians used chaparral to treat ailments from the common cold to snakebites. In recent decades, the herb has been formulated into teas, capsules and tablets, with claims that it can cure a variety of diseases, including cancer.

Researchers believe a chemical in chaparral called nordihydroguaiaretic acid may prevent the replication of cancer cells, as well as viruses and bacteria. However, studies haven't shown that the herb destroys or prevents cancer, and research suggests it can lead to irreversible liver failure.

Shark cartilage. Researchers believe shark cartilage contains a protein that inhibits the formation of new blood

Cancer help or hype?

Dietary supplements are just one form of unconventional treatment for cancer. Other practices include:

Chelation therapy. In chelation, a doctor injects a substance into your bloodstream that binds certain molecules so that they can be removed from your system. This is an approved procedure for heavy-metal toxicity — removing elements such as lead and mercury — but there's no evidence that chelation can treat other diseases, including cancer. The therapy can produce significant side effects, including kidney and bone marrow damage, an irregular heart rhythm, and severe inflammation of the veins. It should only be performed by a knowledgeable doctor.

Macrobiotics. The philosophy behind macrobiotics is that natural foods, utensils and fabrics, combined with a positive attitude and social interconnectedness, promote health and harmony and fight disease, including cancer. However, there's no evidence that macrobiotics prevents or cures cancer. The diet itself has many health benefits, including being low in fat and high in certain vitamins, minerals and phytochemicals. It may be deficient in other nutrients, though, and may require supplemental nutrients to balance its shortcomings.

vessels in tumors, preventing cancer in sharks. Therefore, some people believe that capsules containing shark cartilage can do the same thing in humans — stopping and shrinking cancer. But in limited studies, shark cartilage supplements have generally been found to be ineffective.

Among other things, it's doubtful that the capsules contain enough purified protein to have an effect. Also, you may digest the protein, just as you do other proteins, so it may never get to your bloodstream to be of help. In addition to bad taste, high doses of shark cartilage produce nausea in some people.

Knowing the risks

Unlike prescription medications, the Food and Drug Administration (FDA) doesn't regulate the effectiveness of dietary supplements. In addition, regulations regarding the safety of these products differ from those of the FDA.

With prescription drugs, the manufacturer must prove that the benefits of the drug outweigh any safety concerns before the drug is approved for sale. With dietary supplements, health officials assume the products are safe until they're proved otherwise. Only when a supplement is shown to be unsafe is it removed from the market.

Because dietary supplements are not subject to the same safety procedures as prescription drugs, they can contain toxic substances that may not be listed on the label.

For example, PC SPES was an herbal mixture marketed for the treatment of prostate cancer. Laboratory analysis discovered that several batches of PC SPES were contaminated with pharmaceutical drugs, including an estrogen preparation and the blood thinner warfarin — both of which can be harmful to some people if taken improperly.

The manufacturer voluntarily pulled the product from the market in 2002.

In general, it's wise to avoid dietary supplements if:

- You're having surgery. Supplements may interfere with anesthesia or cause dangerous complications such as bleeding or high blood pressure.
- You're younger than 18 or older than 65. Few supplements have been tested on children. Older adults may metabolize medications differently.
- You're taking prescription or non-prescription medications. Some herbs can cause serious side effects when mixed with certain medications such as aspirin.

Mind-body therapies

These practices are based on the inter-relationship of the mind and body, and the power of one to affect the other. The therapies include hypnosis, meditation and yoga. Mind-body therapies are most commonly used to relieve anxiety and stress and to promote an overall sense of well-being. Some evidence shows that they may also strengthen your immune system.

Mind-body therapies can't cure prostate disease, but some people find them helpful in coping with the emotional and physical effects of cancer, including pain.

Humor therapy

Humor therapy is based on the belief that frequent periods of laughter help distract your attention from health problems. Laughter is also a kind of analgesic — it promotes the release of chemicals that fight pain, as well as reduce depression. The therapy simply involves lightening your day by setting aside time to watch a funny movie or call a friend who makes you laugh.

Hypnosis

People have been using hypnosis to promote healing since ancient times. The therapy may offer relief to those with pain associated with a number of diseases, including cancer. It's also used in treating stress, anxiety and various behavioral disorders.

Hypnosis produces an induced state of relaxation in which your mind stays focused and open to suggestion. During a session, you receive suggestions designed to increase your ability to cope with your condition. This technique can effectively relieve some chronic pain, and it may also reduce nausea and vomiting in people with cancer.

Research indicates that some individuals are more susceptible to hypnotism than are others. Unlike the situations sometimes portrayed in movies and on television, you can't be forced under hypnosis to do something you normally wouldn't want to do. Since it poses little risk of harmful side effects, the therapy may be worth a try.

Meditation

Meditation is a way to calm your mind and body, originating in ancient religious and cultural traditions. In meditation, you focus attention on your breathing, or on repeating a word or sound. This suspends the stream of thoughts that normally occupies your conscious mind, leading to a state of physical relaxation, mental calmness, alertness and psychological balance.

Regular meditation may be used to treat anxiety, stress, pain, depression and insomnia. Studies suggest it may also help reduce blood pressure. The therapy is generally considered safe so long as it doesn't lead to a delay in getting medical attention for an emerging or existing health problem.

Although meditation may sound simple, learning to control your thoughts isn't easy. The more you practice, though, the easier it gets to concentrate without having your mind wander.

Music, dance and art therapy

One or more of these creative expressions can calm and soothe you, revive your spirits, and in some cases, ease pain and suffering. In addition, they help promote self-confidence and may reduce symptoms of depression.

You don't have to be an accomplished dancer, artist or musician to take part — for example, anyone can listen to and enjoy music. Several national organizations promote the use of music, dance and art for health and healing, with chapters set up across the country. Some medical centers also offer music, dance or art therapy programs.

Yoga

The practice of yoga has been around for thousands of years and is rapidly gaining popularity in the United States. This series of postures, along with con-

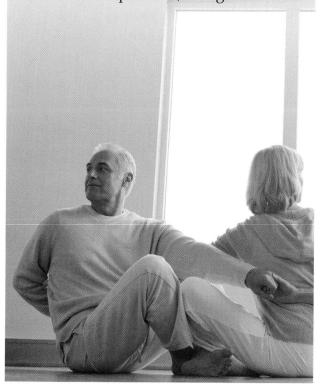

trolled breathing exercises, helps focus your mind less on the concerns of your day and more on the moment as you move your body through poses that require balance and concentration.

According to the National Institutes of Health, yoga can help reduce stress and anxiety, slow breathing, lower blood pressure, and may also decrease symptoms of back pain. However, to be effective, yoga requires training and regular practice.

Tai chi

Tai chi (TIE-chee) is sometimes described as "meditation in motion." Originally developed in China for self-defense, this graceful form of exercise is becoming increasingly integrated into conventional health care around the world. The benefits of tai chi include stress reduction, increased energy and stamina, and greater balance and flexibility — especially for older adults.

Tai chi involves a series of gentle, deliberate postures or movements, with each motion flowing into the next without pause. It's self-paced and non-competitive, and has virtually no negative side effects.

Energy therapies

Some complementary and alternative therapies center on the belief that natural energy forces play an important role in overall health and healing. When an energy pathway in the body becomes blocked or disturbed, illness results. To heal the body, free flow of energy needs to be restored.

There's no proof that these therapies can treat prostate disease, but they do appear to be safe, and they may provide other health benefits.

Acupuncture

Acupuncture is one of the most studied nontraditional medical practices. The National Institutes of Health has issued a consensus statement with evidence that acupuncture helps relieve pain — including pain related to endoscopic procedures and certain forms of chronic pain. Clinical studies have shown that acupuncture is effective in reducing pain in people with cancer. There's stronger evidence that the procedure relieves nausea and vomiting caused by chemotherapy and anesthesia.

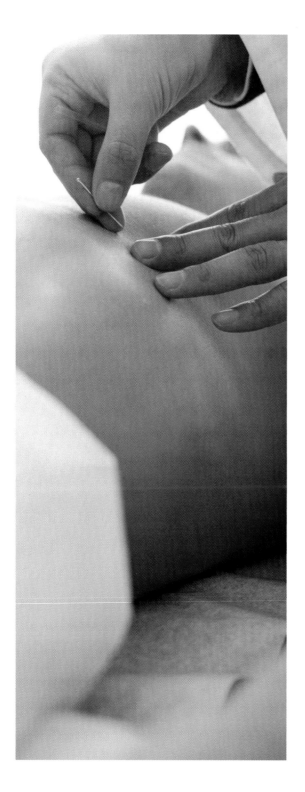

During a typical acupuncture session, a practitioner inserts hair-thin needles into your skin in various combinations. The purpose of the needles is to remove blockages and promote the free flow of life energy (chi). The practitioner may gently move the needles or apply electrical stimulation or heat to them.

Therapy usually involves a series of weekly or biweekly treatments — a typical visit often lasts 30 to 60 minutes. Inserting the needles should cause little or no pain. Some people even find the procedure relaxing. Adverse side effects from acupuncture are rare, but can occur. Make sure your acupuncturist is trained and follows good hygienic practices, including the use of disposable needles.

Acupressure

Acupressure, like acupuncture, stems from the belief that just below your skin are invisible pathways of energy — your body's "life force." During acupressure, a practitioner applies pressure with the fingertips to specific points on your body to restore the free flow of chi and relieve your symptoms. Research on the benefits of acupressure is inconclusive, but some people find the therapy helpful and relaxing.

Other approaches

Some approaches to healing are, in fact, complete medical systems based on traditional practices dating back thousands of years. Treatments focus on prevention and restoring a natural "balance" that enables healing. Studies are limited on the effectiveness of these approaches, and their benefits generally remain unproved.

Ayurveda

This healing philosophy stems from medical practices that originated in India over 5,000 years ago. Ayurveda (i-yur-VA-duh) is based on the principle that mind and body are one and that the body cannot be well if the mind is troubled.

Ayurveda practitioners believe that cancer stems from emotional, spiritual and physical imbalances in life. To treat your cancer, you purge the body of toxic substances through bloodletting, vomiting or bowel emptying. Diet, breathing exercises and massage help rebuild the proper balance. There's no evidence that this practice can cure disease.

Homeopathy

Homeopathic medicine uses highly diluted preparations of natural substances, typically plants and minerals, to treat symptoms of illness. The system is based on a "law of similars." Practitioners believe that if a large dose of a substance causes you to have certain symptoms when you're healthy, a small dose of the same substance can relieve those symptoms.

From a list of nearly 2,000 substances, a homeopath prepares the most appropriate remedy for your set of symptoms. Conditions, such as arthritis, asthma, allergies, colds and influenza are the main reasons why people use this approach. However, scientific research has been unable to confirm whether or not homeopathic medicines can work or explain how they might work.

Naturopathy

This system is based on the healing power of nature. It relies on natural remedies such as sunlight, air and water, combined with supplements, to strengthen the body's healing ability.

Much of the advice of naturopaths is worth heeding: Exercise regularly, practice good nutrition, quit smoking and enjoy nature. However, claims that treatments such as hydrotherapy can detoxify the body and strengthen the immune system aren't backed up by scientific research. There's no evidence that naturopathy can cure cancer or any other disease, as some proponents claim.

Protecting yourself

It's becoming increasingly evident that complementary and alternative medicine can play a role in better health. But it's important to remember some of the differences between these nontraditional approaches and more conventional treatments, some of which have been described in this chapter.

If you decide to try complementary and alternative treatments, protect your health — and your wallet — by learning all you can about the treatments and what benefits their practitioners claim they provide.

The National Center for Complementary and Alternative Medicine (NCCAM) recommends the following steps:

Research the safety and effectiveness of a therapy. The benefits you receive from a treatment should outweigh its risks. To find out more about a therapy, you can request information from the NCCAM, or visit its Web site. You can also search for scientific literature at a public or university library, or via the Internet. Be aware that many Web sites that tout health information are merely advertising fronts for various products.

Determine the skill and reliability of a practitioner. If you're working with a licensed practitioner, check with your local and state medical boards for information about the person's credentials and whether any complaints have been filed against that person. If you're buying a product from a business, check with your local or state business bureau to find out whether any complaints have been filed against the company.

Estimate the total cost of a treatment. Because many complementary and alternative approaches aren't covered by health insurance, it's important to know exactly how much the treatment will cost you.

Talk with your doctor. Your doctor can help you determine whether the treatment may be beneficial and if it's safe.

Too good to be true?

The Food and Drug Administration and the National Council Against Health Fraud recommend that you watch for use of the following practices. These are often warning signs of potentially fraudulent products or therapies:

- The advertisements or promotional materials that include words such as *breakthrough, magical* or *new discovery.* If the product or therapy were in fact a cure, it would be widely reported in the media and your doctor would recommend its use.
- The product materials include pseudo medical jargon such as *detoxify, purify* or *energize.* Such descriptions are difficult to define and measure.
- The manufacturer claims the product can treat a wide range of symptoms, or cure or prevent a number of diseases. No single product can do this.
- The product seems to be backed by scientific studies, but references for these research studies are not provided, are very limited, or are out of date. Manufacturers of legitimate products like to promote the results of scientific studies, not hide them.
- The product has no negative side effects, only benefits. Most medications and other therapies have some side effects.
- The manufacturer of the product accuses the government, medical profession or drug companies of suppressing important information about the helpfulness of the product. There's no reason for the government or medical profession to do so.

Some complementary and alternative therapies may interfere with medications you're taking or adversely affect other health conditions you have.

Don't substitute a proven treatment for an unproven one. If it has been proved that medication, surgery or another treatment recommended by your doctor can help your condition, don't replace this treatment with alternative products, practices or therapies that haven't been proven effective.

Taking responsibility

Good health doesn't just happen. It generally stems from wise decisions you make, such as avoiding smoking, limiting alcohol use, controlling stress and practicing safe sexual habits. Good prostate health can be a part of this overall effort.

It's true that you have no control over or can't change certain aspects about the prostate. But you can be aware of any changes or concerns. Regularly seeing your doctor and having an annual prostate examination increase

your chance of identifying prostate problems early — when it's more likely they can be treated and cured.

The choices you make day in and day out may keep your prostate healthy — or help it to become healthy again. This may require lifestyle changes, such as eating a more nutritious diet and increasing your level of physical activity. Discuss complementary and alternative therapies with your doctor to reduce the risk of potentially dangerous side effects from questionable products or practices.

It's all about taking responsibility for your own well-being. The fact that you're reading this book is an important first step in this process, and an indication that you want to make the right decisions for treating or preventing prostate disease.

Additional resources

Contact these organizations for more information about prostate health, as well as your concerns about prostatitis, BPH and prostate cancer. Some groups offer free printed materials or videos. Others have publications or videos you can purchase.

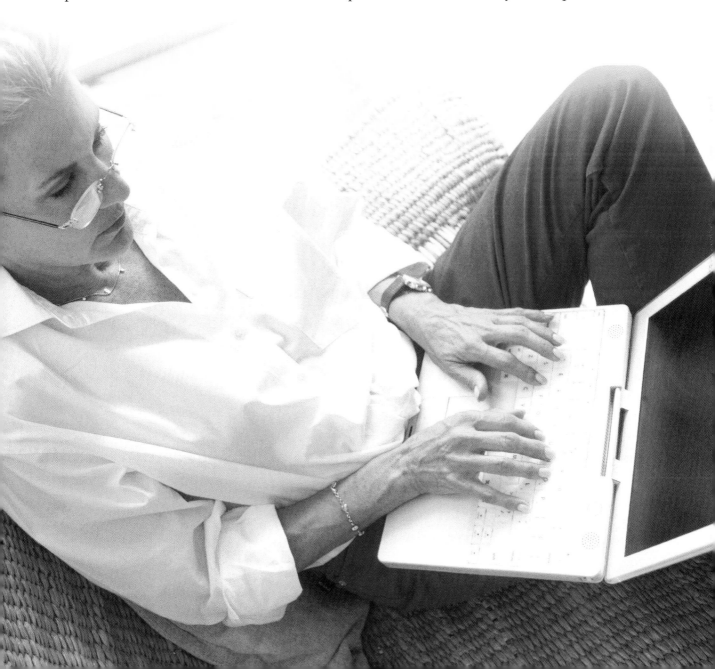

American Cancer Society
1599 Clifton Road NE
Atlanta, GA 30329-4251
404-320-3333 or 800-227-2345
www.cancer.org

American College of Radiology
1891 Preston White Drive
Reston, VA 20191
703-648-8900
www.acr.org

**American Institute
for Cancer Research**
1759 R St. NW
Washington, D.C. 20009
202-328-7744 or 800-843-8114
www.aicr.org

American Prostate Society
P.O. Box 870
Hanover, MD 21076
410-859-3735
www.americanprostatesociety.com

American Urological Association
1000 Corporate Blvd.
Linthicum, MD 21090
410-689-3700 or 866-746-4282
www.auanet.org

Useful information can also be found
at two Web sites sponsored by the
American Urological Association:
• American Urological Association
  Foundation (*www.auafoundation.org*)
• Urology Health
  (*www.urologyhealth.org*)

Cancer Care
275 Seventh Ave., Floor 22
New York, NY 10001
212-712-8400 or 800-813-4673
www.cancercare.org

Cancer Research Institute
1 Exchange Plaza
55 Broadway, Suite 1802
New York, NY 10006
212-688-7515 or 800-992-2623
www.cancerresearch.org

**Centers for Disease
Control and Prevention**
1600 Clifton Road
Atlanta, GA 30333
800-232-4636
www.cdc.gov

**International Foundation for
Functional Gastrointestinal Disorders**
P.O. Box 170864
Milwaukee, WI 53217-8076
414-964-7199 or 888-964-2001
www.iffgd.org

MayoClinic.com
200 1st St. SW
Rochester, MN 55905
www.MayoClinic.com

National Association for Continence
P.O. Box 1019
Charleston, SC 29402-1019
843-377-0900 or 800-252-3337
www.nafc.org

National Cancer Institute
Public Inquiries Office
6116 Executive Blvd., Room 3036A
Bethesda, MD 20892-8322
800-422-6237
www.cancer.gov

**National Center for Complementary
and Alternative Medicine**
NCCAM Clearinghouse
P.O. Box 7923
Gaithersburg, MD 20898
888-644-6226
www.nccam.nih.gov

**National Coalition
of Cancer Survivorship**
1010 Wayne Ave., Suite 770
Silver Spring, MD 20910
301-650-9127 or 888-650-9127
www.canceradvocacy.org

**National Comprehensive
Cancer Network**
275 Commerce Drive, Suite 300
Fort Washington, PA 19034
215-690-0300
www.nccn.org

**National Hospice and
Palliative Care Organization**
1700 Diagonal Road, Suite 625
Alexandria, VA 22314
703-837-1500 or 800-658-8898
www.nhpco.org

National Hospice Foundation
1700 Diagonal Road, Suite 625
Alexandria, VA 22314
703-516-4928
www.nationalhospicefoundation.org

**National Institutes of Health:
Clinical Trials**
9000 Rockville Pike
Bethesda, MD 20892
301-496-4000
www.clinicaltrials.gov

**National Kidney and Urologic
Diseases Information Clearinghouse**
3 Information Way
Bethesda, MD 20892-3580
800-891-5390
www.kidney.niddk.nih.gov

**Natural Medicines
Comprehensive Database**
3120 W. March Lane
Stockton, CA 95208
209-472-2244
www.naturaldatabase.com

Prostate Cancer Foundation
1250 Fourth St.
Santa Monica, CA 90401
310-570-4700 or 800-757-2873
www.prostatecancerfoundation.org

**Radiological Society
of North America**
820 Jorie Blvd.
Oak Brook, IL 60523-2251
630-571-2670 or 800-381-6660
www.rsna.org

**Centers for Medicare &
Medicaid Services**
State Health Insurance Assistance
Program (SHIP)
7500 Security Blvd.
Baltimore, MD 21244-1850
800-633-4227
www.medicare.gov

Us Too International
5003 Fairview Ave.
Downers Grove, IL 60515
630-795-1002 or 800-808-7866
www.ustoo.com

Glossary

A

androgen. A hormone, such as testosterone, that is responsible for the development of male sex organs and other male features, such as facial hair and musculature.

anti-androgen therapy. Medications that prevent the testosterone produced in adrenal glands from reaching prostate cancer cells.

anticholinergic drug. A class of medications that relax the muscles of an overactive bladder, helping to control symptoms of BPH.

antioxidant. A substance found in many vegetables and fruits that may protect body cells from the damaging effects of free radicals. Damage to the prostate from free radicals may cause cancer.

apoptosis. Programmed cell death, which helps keep normal cell growth balanced, and destroys abnormal cells. In cancer cells, this mechanism is disrupted and the cells live longer than normal.

B

benign prostatic hyperplasia (BPH). A noncancerous condition that results when tissue in the interior of the prostate gland enlarges and presses on the urethra, narrowing the channel and restricting the normal flow of urine.

biopsy. A standard diagnostic procedure in which a doctor removes a tiny sample of tissue from your body. This sample is examined under a microscope for signs of disease, such as cancer.

bladder. A hollow, expandable organ in your pelvic region that stores urine, which is produced in the kidneys and transported to the bladder via the ureters. Urine exits the bladder through the urethra.

bone scan. A nuclear imaging procedure based on a radioactive solution that's been injected into your bloodstream. The solution migrates to areas of bone activity that may stem from cancer.

brachytherapy. A treatment for prostate cancer that involves implanting small radioactive seeds directly in or nearby the prostate gland. The implantation may be permanent or temporary.

bulking agent. A substance injected into the urethra that puffs up urethral tissue and narrows the opening of your bladder. Bulking agents are used to treat incontinence.

C

catheter. A thin, flexible tube that can be inserted into your body to inject or drain fluid. A catheter inserted through the penis and urethra allows urine to drain from the bladder.

chemotherapy. A treatment for prostate cancer that uses chemicals to destroy the cancer cells. Unfortunately, the chemicals attack healthy cells as well, causing many unpleasant side effects.

chronic pelvic pain. A form of prostatitis with symptoms that involve more than just the prostate, and are spread throughout the entire pelvic region. This syndrome is difficult to treat because the cause or causes of the pain are unclear.

clinical staging. A series of tests that are done to discover the full extent of cancer in your body — both at its site of origin and its spread to other parts of the body. Also called staging.

complementary and alternative therapies. A broad range of healing philosophies, approaches and techniques that often lie outside conventional medical practice.

computerized tomography (CT). A procedure that uses X-rays to create cross-sectional images of your body's interior with a greater degree of detail and clarity than standard X-rays can provide. A CT scan can locate prostate infections, obstructions and cancer.

cryotherapy. A procedure in which the doctor inserts freezing probes into an organ, such as the prostate gland. Argon gas is used to freeze and kill the abnormal cells. Also called freeze therapy.

cystitis. Inflammation of the bladder, often due to infection. Cystitis can lead to painful urination.

cystoscopy. A procedure that uses a flexible tube equipped with a lens and a light, which can be threaded into your body. For example, the procedure provides clear images of the urethra and bladder that may help your doctor understand what's obstructing your urine flow.

D

digital rectal examination (DRE). A diagnostic procedure in which a doctor inserts a gloved finger into your rectum to feel the prostate. A prostate that feels abnormal to the touch may indicate an infection, enlargement or cancer.

dysuria. A painful, burning discharge of urine, often as a result of inflammation or infection in the bladder.

E

ejaculation. The release of semen through the penis that occurs during male orgasm. This function may be affected by prostate problems or as a side effect of treatment.

erectile dysfunction. The inability to maintain a firm erection of the penis during sexual intercourse. This may be a problem when pelvic nerves are damaged during prostate surgery, radiation therapy or cryotherapy. Sometimes called impotence.

estrogen. A hormone, produced primarily in females but also in males, that helps the body develop feminine physical characteristics. As a medication for prostate cancer, estrogen may be used to block the activity of testosterone.

external beam radiotherapy (EBR). A procedure that directs a concentrated beam of high-energy radiation from a device outside your body to kill cancer cells in your prostate. Intensity-modulated and proton beam are two types of EBR.

G

Gleason grading system. A system to describe the aggressiveness of prostate cancer, named for the system's creator, Donald Gleason, M.D. The system is a scale that goes from 1 to 5, with 1 being the least aggressive form of cancer.

gynecomastia. Excessive growth of male breasts due to lack of the sex hormone testosterone. This is sometimes a side effect of androgen deprivation therapy.

H

heat therapy (thermotherapy). Treatments for BPH that use computer-controlled heat to destroy excess prostate tissue. Different forms use microwaves, high-frequency radio waves and lasers.

hematospermia. The presence of blood in the semen.

hematuria. The presence of blood in the urine.

holmium laser enucleation of the prostate (HoLEP). A surgical procedure that uses a special high-energy, low-penetration laser to provide relief from the symptoms of BPH. Excess prostate tissue is cut out and pushed into the bladder, where a special device grinds it into finer pieces and sucks it out through the cystoscope.

hormone. A chemical messenger secreted by one of the endocrine glands and carried through the bloodstream. Hormones help regulate many body functions, including digestion, metabolism and reproduction. They may play a role in the development of prostate cancer.

hormone therapy. Treatment with drugs or surgery that reduces the supply of male sex hormones such as testosterone — which can stimulate prostate cancer cells. Another form of this treatment blocks hormones from reaching the cancer. Also called hormone deprivation therapy or androgen deprivation therapy (ADT).

I

impotence. The inability to maintain a firm erection during sexual intercourse. *See* erectile dysfunction.

incontinence (urinary). The inability to control the release of urine, which may be an often temporary side effect of prostate treatment.

indolent. Describes the stage of a disease, such as cancer, when it develops slowly and produces few symptoms.

intensity-modulated radiation therapy (IMRT). A form of external beam radiotherapy that uses high-powered X-rays to kill cancer cells in the prostate gland.

international prostate symptoms score (IPSS). A series of standardized questions that help you and your doctor determine how prostate symptoms are affecting you and guide decisions on how you should be treated.

interstitial laser therapy (ILT). A form of heat therapy for BPH that uses a fiber-optic device to direct laser energy into the interior of the prostate and destroy excess tissue that's obstructing urinary flow.

K

Kegel exercises. Voluntary movements of your pelvic floor muscles to improve their strength and tone. Kegel exercises can help to reduce mild to moderate incontinence.

L

laparoscopy. Surgery to examine the inside of your abdomen with a laparoscope and remove lymph nodes from your pelvic area that are suspected of being cancerous. A laparoscope is a thin, lighted tube containing a fiber-optic camera.

latent. Describes the stage of a disease, such as cancer, when it is present in your body but inactive, producing no symptoms.

LH-RH agonist. A medication for prostate cancer that interrupts the activity of the LH-RH hormone (see entry below). As a result, your testicles never get the message to produce testosterone.

luteinizing hormone-releasing hormone (LH-RH). A hormone that alerts the pituitary gland to release luteinizing hormone (LH). In turn, LH signals your testicles to make testosterone, which stimulates prostate cancer cells.

lymph node biopsy. A procedure to remove tissue from the lymph nodes so that the samples can be examined for signs of cancer.

lymph nodes. Small, bean-shaped structures located throughout your body that are critical to your immune system. They store special cells that help protect you from bacteria and other organisms.

M

magnetic resonance imaging (MRI). Imaging procedure that uses magnetic fields to produce detailed pictures of your body' interior.

maximum androgen blockade. Treatment designed to stop your body from producing male hormones. This treatment can include hormone medications, surgery to remove the testicles, or both.

metastasis. The spread of disease-producing agents, such as cancer or bacteria, from one location in the body to another location.

metastatic prostate cancer. Abnormal cell growth that has spread outside the prostate to tissue in the lymph nodes, bones and other organs in your body.

mutation. A change or alteration in cell DNA. Sometimes, this change has no effect or can improve the organism, and other times it can hurt the organism.

N

needle biopsy. A procedure in which a surgeon inserts a small needle into an organ, such as the prostate gland. Using the needle, the surgeon removes tiny samples of tissue, which are examined in a laboratory for signs of cancer.

O

open prostatectomy. Surgery to remove internal tissue of the prostate that's obstructing the urethra. The procedure may be used to relieve severe symptoms of BPH.

orchiectomy. Surgery to remove the testicles, which prevents the production of testosterone. Hormone-blocking drugs have reduced the need for this form of surgery. Also called castration.

P

palpable tumor. An abnormal growth of tissue that can be felt, or palpated — for example, during a digital rectal exam.

peripheral zone. One of the zones of the prostate located on the outer edge of the organ. Very often if there's prostate cancer, it will develop first in the peripheral zone.

pelvic floor muscles. A layer of strong muscle tissue in the lower part of your pelvis that helps control bladder function and bowel movements.

pelvic lymph node dissection. A procedure to remove lymph nodes located near the prostate. A pathologist will examine the tissue in a laboratory to discover whether prostate cancer has spread.

perineal prostatectomy. A procedure in which a surgeon makes an incision in the perineum to remove the prostate gland. In a man, the perineum is the space between the scrotum and the anus.

photosensitive vaporization of the prostate (PVP). A surgical procedure that uses a high-energy laser to relieve symptoms of BPH. The procedure is also known as Greenlight PV. Most prostates can be treated with PVP, although very large prostates may have to be done in two separate operations.

proctitis. An inflamed rectum, often occurring with bleeding, diarrhea and pain.

prostate gland. An organ that's located just below a man's bladder and surrounds the top of the urethra. This gland produces most of the fluids in semen.

prostate-specific antigen (PSA). A protein produced by the prostate gland that's a vital component of semen. A PSA test can determine how much of this protein is circulating in your blood. PSA comes in two forms — that which is bound to blood proteins, and that which is unbound, called free PSA.

prostatic intraepithelial neoplasia (PIN). Abnormal prostate cells found in biopsies that may signal an increased chance that cancer will develop. PIN samples are usually classified as high grade, indicating the level of risk.

prostatic stent. A tiny metal coil that is inserted into the urethra. When in place, the stent expands to widen the urethra and keep it open.

prostatitis. A general term for inflammation of the prostate gland. The condition encompasses four distinct categories.

R

radiation oncologist. A specialist in cancer treatment who performs radiation therapy.

radiation therapy. The use of radiation — with either an external beam or internal implants or seeds — to kill cancer cells.

radical prostatectomy. A procedure in which a surgeon removes your entire prostate gland, usually along with nearby tissue. Depending on where the incision is made, the surgery may be retropubic (in the lower abdomen) or perineal (between the anus and scrotum).

radioactive seed implant. *See* brachytherapy.

rectum. The final section of the large intestine, which stores solid waste until you're ready to go to the bathroom. The waste exits through the anal canal. A physician feels the inner wall of your rectum, which lies next to the prostate, to check for tumors and other abnormalities.

resectoscope. A thin tubular device containing a sliding knife or electrified wire, which can be used for certain surgical procedures of the prostate.

robotic-assisted laparoscopic radical prostatectomy (RALRP). A surgical procedure for prostate cancer in which all instruments are controlled by a mechanical device guided by the surgeon from a computer console, based on the principles of laparoscopic surgery.

S

semen. A thick, whitish fluid containing sperm cells. Men discharge this fluid from the penis during ejaculation.

seminal vesicles. Sac-like glands located behind the bladder in men that store and produce most of the ejaculatory fluid in semen. Removal of these structures may occur during prostate cancer treatment.

sperm. Male reproductive cells that are produced in the testicles and transmitted in semen.

sphincter. A ring of muscle fiber that opens and contracts to control the release of urine from the bladder. There are actually two sphincters: an internal sphincter that encircles the bladder opening to the urethra, and an external sphincter, located just below the prostate.

staging. *See* clinical staging.

surgical margins. The borders of tissue that's cut and removed during surgery. One goal of prostate cancer surgery is to remove the prostate gland in a way that leaves behind tissue edges (margins) that are free of cancer.

T

testicles. The egg-shaped glands in the scrotum that produce sperm as well as testosterone.

testosterone. A sex hormone manufactured in the testicles that produces male sexual characteristics.

This hormone is an androgen that can stimulate the growth of prostate cancer.

three-dimensional conformal radiation therapy (3D-CRT). Radiation therapy that uses computer software to produce three-dimensional images of an organ, such as the prostate gland. These images allow a therapist to direct radiation beams so that they correspond to the shape of the organ — sparing normal tissue located nearby from damage.

TNM rating system. A method for describing the spread of cancer. *T* stands for "tumor" and signifies the extent of the cancer in, and adjacent to, the prostate gland. *N* stands for "nodes" and signifies whether the cancer has spread to nearby lymph nodes. *M* stands for "metastasis" — cancer that has spread to other tissues or organs.

transitional zone. One of the zones of the prostate. This internal zone surrounds the urethra and is often the part of the prostate that enlarges in older adults to cause BPH.

transrectal ultrasonography (TRUS). The use of sound waves that are bounced off the prostate and converted by a computer into an image of the prostate.

transurethral vaporization of the prostate (TUVP). A form of heat therapy involving a metal instrument that emits a high-frequency electrical current. A doctor uses this instrument to remove excess tissue from the prostate when treating BPH.

transurethral incision of the prostate (TUIP). A procedure in which a surgeon makes several small incisions in the prostate gland and bladder neck. These cuts allow the urethra to expand, making it easier to urinate.

transurethral microwave therapy (TUMT). A form of heat therapy that uses microwave energy to destroy internal tissue in an enlarged prostate gland that may be obstructing the urethra.

transurethral needle ablation (TUNA). A form of heat therapy that directs radio waves through needles that are inserted into the prostate gland. This energy destroys excess tissue in the prostate that is obstructing the urethra and blocking urine flow.

transurethral resection of the prostate (TURP). A procedure in which a surgeon threads a resectoscope into the urethra and cuts away excess prostate tissue. TURP has the longest history of successful relief of BPH symptoms in men with enlarged prostate glands or the most bothersome symptoms.

tumor. An abnormal growth of tissue. The growth may be cancerous (malignant) or not cancerous (benign).

tumor markers. Substances circulating in the blood that are produced by tumors. The amount of a tumor marker in circulation may reflect the extent of the tumor.

U

ultrasonography. An imaging technique that uses the echoes of sound waves directed into the body to create an image of its internal structures. A transrectal ultrasound is frequently used for diagnosing prostate problems.

ureters. The tubes that carry urine from your kidneys to your bladder.

urethra. The tube extending from the bladder to the tip of the penis. The urethra carries urine from the bladder. During ejaculation, the urethra also transports semen from the prostate gland.

urologist. A doctor who specializes in treating disorders of the urinary and reproductive systems in men.

V

vasa deferentia. Two tubes that carry sperm from the testicles to the prostate gland and urethra. These will be severed during a prostatectomy.

visual laser ablation of the prostate (VLAP). A treatment that applies laser energy to dry up and destroy excess cells in the prostate gland.

W

watchful waiting. The decision to hold off on aggressive treatment and observe your condition to see if it changes.

Index

A

ABCD staging system, 120
abdominal exercises, 225
absorbent pads, 171–172
acupressure, 240
acupuncture, 239–240
acute bacterial prostatitis (category 1)
    defined, 55
    problems, 55–56
    signs and symptoms, 55
ADT. *See* androgen deprivation therapy
advanced cancer. *See* metastatic prostate
      cancer
aerobic exercise, 221–222
African wild potato, 233
age
    BPH treatments and, 101
    prostate cancer treatments and, 145
    prostate changes based on, 207
    prostate problems and, 25
    as risk factor, 20, 25
alcohol
    heavy consumption, 216–217
    limiting, 83
    prostate disease and, 230
alcohol ablation, 97
alfuzosin (Uroxatral), 84
alpha blockers
    blood pressure and, 84–85
    for BPH, 84–85
    FDA approved, 84
    side effects, 84
    for urine flow, 64
alprostadil
    defined, 174
    intraurethral therapy, 175–176
    needle-injection therapy, 174, 175

American Cancer Society (ACS), 34, 35,
    203, 246
American College of Radiology, 246
American Institute for Cancer Research,
    246
American Medical Association (AMA),
    prostate screening, 34–35
American Prostate Society, 246
Americans With Disabilities Act, 196–198
American Urological Association (AUA),
    34, 35
    contact information, 246
    Symptom Index, 73–76
androgen deprivation therapy (ADT)
    anti-androgens, 152
    benefits, 153
    candidates, 153
    defined, 150
    in early-stage cancers, 151
    intermittent use of drugs, 152–153
    luteinizing hormone-releasing hormone
      (LH-RH), 151
    lymph nodes and, 151
    risks, 153
angiogenesis inhibitors, 143
anti-androgens, 152
antibiotics, for prostatitis, 61–64
anticholinergics, 86, 169
antihistamines, 83
anxiety, 58–59, 183
appetite, stimulating, 195–196
arm curl, 225
artificial sphincter, 170, 171
aspirin, 124
asymptomatic inflammatory prostatitis, 59
atypical small acinar proliferation (ASAP),
    112
ayurveda, 241

cryotherapy
    candidates, 142
    defined, 141
    potential problems, 142
    procedure, 141–142, 158
CT. *See* computerized tomography
cystography, 166
cystometrography, 166
cystometry, 77
cystoscopy
    defined, 40, 166
    procedure, 77–78
    uses, 40

D

dairy products, 212, 216
darifenacin (Enablex), 86, 169
decision tree
    BPH, 78, 79
    prostate cancer, 121
decongestants, 83
deep breathing, 188
depression, 184
DHEA (dehydroepiandrosterone), 23
diarrhea
    causes, 178
    curbing, 194
    water/salt loss, 179
diet
    as risk factor, 22–23
    See also eating; foods
dietary supplements, 233–236
    African wild potato, 233
    cancer fighters, 234–235
    chaparral, 234
    derivation of, 233
    pumpkin seeds, 233
    pygeum, 99, 233
    risks, 236
    rye grass, 233
    saw palmetto, 233–234
    stinging nettle, 233
    types of, 233
    See also complementary and
        alternative therapies (CAM)

digital rectal examination (DRE)
    BPH and, 73
    BPH detection and, 27
    defined, 26
    illustrated, 26
    prostate cancer detection and, 27
    prostatitis detection and, 27
    PSA test with, 28
    recommendation, 27
    statistics, 27
diuretics, limiting, 83
docetaxel (Taxotere), 156
doctors
    in complementary and alternative
        therapies consideration,
        242–244
    experience, 103, 229
    questions for, 143, 182
    search, 146–147
    seeing regularly, 229
doxazosin (Cardura), 84
DRE. *See* digital rectal examination
dutasteride (Avodart), 33, 85
dynamic contrast-enhanced (DCE)
    images, 47

E

early prostate cancer antigen 2 (EPCA-2),
    37
eating
    appetite stimulation, 195–196
    calories, increasing, 192
    drinking and, 196
    nutritional drinks, 193–195
    prepared meals, 195
    protein intake, 193
    See also foods
ejaculation, PSA tests and, 30–31
emotional timetable, 198–200
emotions
    anxiety, 183
    coping strategies, 185–189
    depression, 184
    expectations, 183–185
    sense of loss, 184–185

friends
    reaching out to, 200
    well-meaning, 198
friendship, support groups, 203
fruits, 213–214

G

garlic, 212
gene research, 37
gene therapy, 157
Gleason grading scale
    defined, 113
    grades, 113
    scores, 114
grading cancer, 112–114
green tea, 211
guided imagery, 188

H

heat therapies
    defined, 86
    laser therapy, 89
    microwave therapy, 87
    as outpatient procedures, 87
    process, 86–87
    radiofrequency therapy, 88–89
help, accepting, 200
herbal therapies
    for BPH, 99
    for prostatitis, 67
holmium laser enucleation of the prostate
        (HoLEP), 94, 95
homeopathy, 241
hormone therapy, 137, 150–153
    benefits, 153
    cancer control, 162
    candidates, 153
    defined, 150
    in early-stage prostate cancers, 151
    intermittent drug use, 152–153
    risks, 153
    testosterone blocking drugs, 152
    testosterone reduction drugs, 151
    voice and appearance effects, 162

human glandular kallikrein, 37
humor therapy, 237
hypnosis, 237

I

imaging techniques
    bone scan, 49
    computerized tomography (CT), 44–45
    cystoscopy, 40
    magnetic resonance imaging (MRI),
        46–47
    nuclear scans, 48
    positron emission tomography (PET),
        48, 50
    types of, 39
    ultrasound, 28, 41
    X-ray, 42
imipramine (Tofranil), 169
immunotherapy, 143, 156–157
impotence
    biopsy and, 124
    erectile dysfunction vs., 180
    risk with retropubic surgery, 129–130
incontinence
    catheters and absorbent pads,
        171–172
    causes, 165
    controlling, 164–172
    defined, 164
    long-term, 164
    Medicare coverage, 180
    medications, 169
    mixed, 167
    overflow, 166
    penile clamps, 172
    prostate cancer surgery and, 132
    stress, 165
    surgery, 169–171
    treatments, 167–172
    types of, 165–167
    urge, 165
infertility, prostatitis and, 68
inflammation, 13
    bacterial infection, 18
    causes, 54

in DRE, 60
    signs and symptoms, 18
    white blood cells indication, 61
    See also prostatitis
integrative medicine, 232
intensity-modulated radiation therapy
        (IMRT), 135–137
    defined, 135
    dosage, 137
    new method, 137
    targeting guides, 136
    treatments, 135–136
International Foundation for Functional
        Gastrointestinal Disorders, 246
international prostate symptom score
        (IPSS), 73
interstitial laser therapy (ILT), 89
intraprostatic injections, 97
intraurethral therapy, 175–176
intravenous pyelogram, 78

K

Kegel exercises, 167–169

L

laser surgery
    defined, 93
    laser types, 93
    photosensitive vaporization of the
        prostate (PVP), 93–94
    transurethral evaporation of the
        prostate (TUEP), 94
    visual laser ablation of the prostate
        (VLAP), 94
laser therapy, 89
lifestyle changes
    for BPH, 83
    prostate cancer and, 181–204
    for prostatitis, 65
living wills, 204
low back stretch, 223
lutein, 208
luteinizing hormone-releasing hormone
        (LH-RH), 151

lycopene, 208
lymph nodes
    biopsy, 116
    removal, 129

M

macrobiotics, 235
magnetic resonance imaging (MRI)
    defined, 46
    images, 46, 47
        for prostate cancer, 116
    uses, 46
    See also imaging techniques
markers, 37
MayoClinic.com, 247
Mayo Clinic Healthy Weight Pyramid, 213,
        214, 217
medical visits, 182–183
medications
    incontinence, 169
    pain, 159–161, 162
medications (BPH)
    alpha blockers, 84–85
    anticholinergics, 86
    combination drug therapy, 85–86
    enzyme inhibitors, 85
    new drug classes, 98
    types of, 83
medications (erectile dysfunction)
    alprostadil, 174–176
    needle-injection therapy, 174–175
    oral, 173–174
medications (prostatitis)
    alpha blockers, 64
    antibiotics, 61–64
    muscle relaxants, 64
    pain relievers, 64
meditation, 237–238
metabolism changes, 49
metastatic prostate cancer
    chemotherapy, 155–156
    defined, 149
    experimental procedures, 156–157
    hormone therapy, 150–155
    options, 150

proton beam, 137–138
radioactive seed implants, 138–140
risks, 141
use of, 135
See also treatments (prostate cancer)
radical prostatectomy, 128
perineal surgery, 130
retropubic surgery, 128–130
robotic surgery, 132–134
radioactive drugs, 158
radioactive seed implants, 138–140
defined, 138
illustrated, 139
movement out of prostate, 148
permanent seeding, 140
procedure, 140
seeds, 138–140
radiofrequency ablation, 161
radiofrequency therapy. *See* transurethral
needle ablation (TUNA)
Radiological Society of North America,
248
recurrence fear, 191, 204
relaxation techniques, 188
reproductive system, 14–18
retrograde ejaculations, 91
retropubic surgery, 128–130
defined, 128
impotence risk, 129–130
lymph node removal, 129
orgasm and, 130
prostate removal, 129, 130
risk factors
age, 20
bone mass, 21
controllable, 21–23
family history, 21
race and ethnicity, 20–21
sexual activity, 21–22
supplemental hormones, 23
uncontrollable, 20–21
robotic-assisted laparoscopic radical
prostatectomy (RALRP)
benefits, 134
defined, 132
illustrated, 133

procedure, 133, 134
risks, 134
See also surgery (for prostate cancer)
rye grass, 233

s

sacral nerve stimulator, 171
saline laxatives, 179
sampling errors, 123
saw palmetto, 68, 99
defined, 233–234
safety, 234
self-care
for body, 185
for fatigue, 190–191
reduction steps, 190
semen, 14
sense of loss, 184–185
sexual activity
BPH surgery and, 102
as chronic pelvic pain cause, 58
as risk factor, 21–22
sexually transmitted diseases (STDs), 21,
24
shark cartilage, 234–235
side effects compensation, 189
sildenafil (Viagra), 173, 174
sitz baths, 67
sleep, 190–191
solifenacin (Vesicare), 86, 169
soy
benefits, 211
sources, 210
See also foods
soy sauce, 230
sphincter, 14–18
spirituality, 186
staging cancer
ABCD system, 120
defined, 117
stage I, 118, 120
stage II, 118, 120
stage III, 119, 120
stage IV, 119, 120
TNM system, 117–120

State Health Insurance Assistance
    Program (SHIP), 248
STDs (sexually transmitted diseases),
    21–22, 24
stenting, 97
stimulant laxatives, 180
stinging nettle, 233
stool softeners, 179
strengthening exercises, 224–225
stress, 58–59, 230
stress incontinence, 165
supplemental hormones, as risk factor, 23
support groups
    benefits, 201, 202–203
    exchange of advice, 202–203
    finding, 203
    friendship, 203
    join decision, 201
    online, 203
    sense of belonging in, 202
    types of, 201
    understanding in, 202
support system, 185
surgery (for BPH)
    decision, 89–90
    holmium laser enucleation of the
        prostate (HoLEP), 94
    laser, 93–94
    mechanical device options, 96–97
    open prostatectomy, 94–96
    recommendation, 89
    recovery, 96
    transurethral incision of the prostate
        (TUIP), 92
    transurethral resection of the prostate
        (TURP), 89, 90–92
    transurethral vaporization of the
        prostate (TUVP), 92
    types, 90
surgery (for incontinence)
    artificial sphincter, 170, 171
    bulking material injections, 170
    sacral nerve stimulator, 171
surgery (for prostate cancer), 128–134
    benefits, 132
    candidates, 132

choices, 128
exercise and sports after, 204
as pain relief strategy, 158
perineal, 130
prostate removal, 129, 130
radical prostatectomy, 128
retropubic, 128–130
risks, 132
testicular, 153–155
surgery (for prostatitis), 67, 68
survival, coping with, 199
sweets, 216

T

tadalafil (Cialis), 173, 174
tai chi, 239
tamsulosin (Flomax), 84
targeted chemotherapy, 143
terazosin (Hytrin), 84
testicular surgery, 153–155
    benefits, 154
    bilateral orchiectomy, 154
    candidates, 154
    defined, 153–154
    risks, 154–155
TNM staging system, 117
tobacco, as risk factor, 23
toe and heel raise, 224
tolterodine (Detrol), 86, 169
tomatoes, 208
tramadol (Ultram), 160–161
transcutaneous electrical nerve stimulation
    (TENS), 158
transrectal biopsy, 111
transrectal ultrasound, 28, 41
transurethral evaporation of the prostate
    (TUEP), 94
transurethral incision of the prostate
    (TUIP), 92
transurethral microwave therapy
    (TUMT), 87–88
    candidates, 88
    defined, 87
    illustrated, 87
    side effects, 88

TUMT. *See* transurethral microwave
    therapy
TUNA. *See* transurethral needle ablation
TURP. *See* transurethral resection of the
    prostate

U

ultrasensitive PSA test, 37
ultrasound
    defined, 28
    images, 41
    procedure, 28, 41
    for prostate cancer, 115
    transrectal, 28, 41
    See also imaging techniques
upper thigh stretch, 223
ureters, 18
urethral stricture, 165
urge incontinence, 165
urinary catheters, 97, 171–172
urinary flow test, 76
urinary system, 18, 55
urinary tract
    examination with cystoscopy, 40
    infections, 31, 60
    prostate tumor symptoms, 109–110
urine samples, 60–61
urine test, 27–28, 73
urodynamic testing, 166
uroflowometry, 166
urologists, when to see, 38
Us Too International, 248

V

vacuum erection devices, 176–177
vardenafil (Levitra), 173, 174
vasa deferentia, 14
vasectomies, 24
vegetables
    cruciferous, 212
    eating, 213–215
visual laser ablation of the prostate
        (VLAP), 94
vitamins, 209

W

walking, 221
wall push-ups, 224
watchful waiting
    advantages, 82, 127
    age and, 126–127
    BPH, 82–83
    candidates, 127
    defined, 82
    lifestyle changes and, 83
    prostate cancer, 126–127
    risks, 82, 127
white blood cells, 61
wide-field radiation, 161
word repetition, 188
work
    adjustments, 196
    continuing, 196–198
    employer accommodations, 198

X

X-ray
    chest, 115
    contrast dye, 42
    defined, 42
    images, 42, 43
    uses, 42
    See also imaging techniques

Y

yoga, 238–239

Z

zinc, 209